Head On

An
All Black's
memoir

Head On

Carl Hayman

HarperCollins*Publishers*

HarperCollins*Publishers*
Australia • Brazil • Canada • France • Germany • Holland • India
Italy • Japan • Mexico • New Zealand • Poland • Spain • Sweden
Switzerland • United Kingdom • United States of America

First published in 2023
by HarperCollins*Publishers* (New Zealand) Limited
Unit D1, 63 Apollo Drive, Rosedale, Auckland 0632, New Zealand
harpercollins.co.nz

A catalogue record for this book is available from the National Library of New Zealand

ISBN 978 1 7755 4235 3 (paperback)
ISBN 978 1 7754 9266 5 (ebook)
ISBN 978 1 4607 4923 4 (audio book)

Cover design by HarperCollins Design Studio
Cover image © PHOTOSPORT
Typeset in Adobe Garamond Pro by Kirby Jones
Printed and bound by CPI Group (UK) Ltd, Croydon, CR0 4YY

This book is dedicated to my children: Sophie, Taylor, Charles and Genevieve.

To everyone that has played a part in my life — friends, family, coaches and supporters — and in particular my late mother who I miss every day, I thank you.

Lastly, to anyone struggling: there is always hope.

CONTENTS

August 19, 2006   1

Prologue: *Rescue III*, Pt I   7

1. Pau, 2016–18, Falling Down   13

2. Oaonui, 1979–92, Growing up   41

3. London, 2020, Diagnosis   55

4. Dunedin, 1993–2000, Southern Man   73

5. Mexico, 2022, The Tourist   95

6. Albany, 2000, All Black #1000   117

7. Makalu, 2019, Head in the Clouds   151

8. Cardiff, 2007, Game Plan Two   162

9. Ōpunake, 2022, My False Friend   193

10. Newcastle, 2007–10, 'Million-dollar' Man   216

11. Taupō, 2020, Ironman   242

12. Toulon, 2010–15, Break Point   252

13. New Plymouth, 2022, Standing Up   277

Epilogue: *Rescue III*, Pt II   295

Afterword   303

Acknowledgements   311

AUGUST 19, 2006

HERE WE GO AGAIN. Scrum time.

My time.

The score is locked at 6–6, midway through the first half. The Bledisloe Cup is on the line. A capacity crowd at Eden Park is in good voice. The Test has been played at a frenetic pace. We've got the upper hand in the forwards, but when we look at one another, we see the same tension each of us feels. These Wallaby backs — George Gregan, Stephen Larkham, Stirling Mortlock, Matt Giteau — are so smart. If their forwards can keep them in the game long enough, they can strike from anywhere.

The scrum is on our 40-metre line. We crouch, engage and hit — our 890 kilograms of muscle and bone smashing into their similarly statured resistance. All 16 men gasp as they take the strain. For a moment, it holds steady. Then it begins to buckle. There's a problem. Our halfback, Byron Kelleher, has yet to get to the scrum with the ball. For fuck's sake. The ref calls the mess off and we disengage. What a useless waste of energy that was.

We go through the whole strange courting ritual that precedes the scrum again. This time it sets and stays. The ball goes in. The scrum holds rock-steady on my tighthead side. More than that, Keven Mealamu, Tony Woodcock and I begin to inch forward, showing clear superiority. We clear our ball easily and the backs are immediately on the front foot.

Job done.

By the time I've disengaged, Dan Carter has already brought Luke McAlister back against the grain to set up a ruck. I fan out to the right, anticipating two or three rucks ahead. After the first ruck, Kelleher flings to Chris Jack, who is hit behind the advantage line. It's okay, though. The ball is released quickly and Carter, our resident genius, is pulling the strings and has called for it on the short side. My side. He dummies and loses a defender before being tackled low by the second man — low enough for him to use his brilliant balance and hands to find his support player.

That's me.

I take the ball and… bang… (fade to black).

I knew nothing about what happened, but today I can look back and see.

I was hit almost immediately by Wycliff Palu, Australia's 120-kilogram bull-in-a-china-shop No. 8. As he went to wrap me up ball-and-all, our heads speared into one another. It'd be a sure-fire red card now, but back then, it was just one of those things. No malice on his part. A bit of bad luck. I crumpled in a heap and momentarily lay prone as the ball was shifted left into Richie McCaw's hands. I got to my hands and knees and then flopped onto my arse. Palu was groggy nearby, on one knee as play carried on. I pushed off the turf with my left hand but couldn't get upright. I stumbled and toppled over again.

Play carried on. We attacked down the left through Joe Rokocoko and made good ground into Australia's half. We were in the ascendancy but two phases later, Jerry Collins attempted a long, cut-out 'hero' pass that Lote Tuqiri read like a children's book and intercepted. He set sail for the tryline, with only one defender between him and glory. That's me. You can see me in the footage, still being treated by our medic, still in la-la land. I watch myself brush off the medic and lurch after Tuqiri. I wince. Even at the best of times, a tighthead prop in the pink of health has got little chance defending one-on-one against one of the world's most dynamic wings. A tighthead prop who has been concussed and is ataxic — one of many medical terms that I've become too familiar with, one which means displaying any of a range of the signs of mental impairment following a concussive brain injury — has no chance. You can guess how that duel went.

They won that battle and scored, but we won the war: the Test match.

I have no memory of the night that followed, but I can't help but think about it now, and speculate.

I was lucky, if you can call it that, in that this was, to the best of my fractured and fading memory, the only big, symptomatic concussion I suffered in my professional rugby career. But how lucky? Knowing what I know now, I can't help but wonder if my future was forever altered that day. A second before the impact with Palu, my brain was floating innocently inside my skull, suspended in the cerebrospinal fluid that acts as a protective cushion between brain and bone. During the impact, however, the whiplash effect pushed the organ through the fluid and into the wall of the skull, damaging neurons and bruising the brain at the site of impact.

Was the complicated chemistry within my brain forever altered in that moment? Did harmful tau protein start collecting in the crevices of my grey matter as a result of this one traumatic event, or were they already gathering as the result of the thousands upon thousands of subconcussive hits I was taking over hundreds of games, hundreds of contact training sessions and untold interactions with unforgiving scrum machines? Was there a point in my career where I could have walked away and remained undamaged?

In the end, it's academic. Because no matter where it started, the sad fact of the matter is that my brain is irreversibly damaged. It will never get better. The best I can hope for is to slow down the deterioration. I certainly can't change the past. I can't fully comprehend my future, either, or perhaps I just don't want to.

I am what I am: a former professional rugby player with early-onset dementia and probable chronic traumatic encephalopathy, a neurodegenerative disease that somehow sounds less sinister when given its popular acronym, CTE. I'm a flawed human being. Like everyone else, I want to be liked and loved, but whether it is because I don't want to burden them with my shit or whether it's just because I'm emotionally broken, I specialise in pushing people away, even the ones who matter most to me.

In part, that's why I'm telling my story. Whether I like it or not, and in more ways than one, I am a living, breathing, suffering cautionary tale.

PROLOGUE

RESCUE III, PT I

IN MY FORTY-FIRST YEAR of shuffling around on this planet, I bought a boat.

Well, *we* bought a boat. But before I introduce you to Kiko Matthews, my partner in our business, Chaddy's Charters, I want you to meet *Rescue III*.

She was built in 1953 as a Liverpool-class, three-skin mahogany-hull lifeboat and was christened the *Tillie Morrison Sheffield II*.

Her namesake, the original *Tillie Morrison*, was a 1947-built carriage-launched, self-righting lifeboat made by J. Samuel White of Cowes at a cost of £10,573. She was gifted to the

Royal National Lifeboat Institution (RNLI) by the Morrison brothers of Sheffield, in remembrance of their sister (for whom she was named), and presented to the people of Bridlington on the Yorkshire coast by HRH The Duchess of Kent, president of the RNLI. The ceremony took place in front of Lord Middleton, Lord Lieutenant of East Riding, Yorkshire, the Archbishop of York, the Right Honourable and Most Reverend Cyril Foster Garbett, and music was performed by the band of the 1st Battalion Duke of Wellington's Regiment. It was quite the do.

When she was moved from Bridlington six years later to the Welsh seaside resort of Llandudno, a replacement was needed. *Tillie Morrison II,* also built in Cowes on the Isle of Wight at the slightly steeper cost of £14,481, was promptly launched. There was the odd lifeboat dignitary at her naming ceremony, but no royalty and the blessing was carried out by the Reverend CE Paterson, the vicar of the Holy Trinity Church in Cowes. There was some controversy over the name. It was proposed the new boat be called *Robert Redhead* but the Morrison brothers, who had donated the original lifeboat, had also bequeathed money in their wills to ensure their sister's name remained on a boat at Bridlington. *Tillie Morrison II* it was, and within a month, she was saving lives.

Yes, *Tillie II* might not have arrived with all the fanfare of her namesake, but by any standards 1953 was a momentous year. It was the year of the late Queen Elizabeth II's coronation, of Joseph Stalin's death and on May 29, our very own Sir Edmund Hillary 'knocked the bastard off'.

The All Blacks set off on a tour to Europe that year, too. Six months later, they returned home, having won 30 of the 36 matches they played, drawn two and lost four, including Tests against Wales and France. It was also the year in which the first clear links between smoking and lung cancer were discovered and it feels important to mention those two things in the same paragraph, even if it might not be immediately clear why.

Tillie Morrison II performed rescues off Bridlington until 1967, when she was relocated to the opposite side of the world. *Tillie* was renamed *Rescue III* and served the Christchurch community faithfully as part of the Sumner Surf Life Saving Club fleet until being retired from active service in 1993.

That year she travelled north to New Plymouth, the largest town in my home province of Taranaki, and ever since has been taking sightseers around the Ngā Motu/Sugar Loaf islands: a collection of five small uninhabited islands and several sea stacks near the port — in the employ of Chaddy's Charters, the business that Kiko and I bought.

That's our happy place, hers and mine: out on the sea around those 1.7-million-year-old remnants of volcanic activity, among the seal colonies and the little blue penguins where, on any given day, you might also see reef heron, whales or dolphins. There's something about the sea air that's reviving.

Even on the most challenging day, I come off the boat feeling better about life.

Rescue III weighs 12 tonnes, has a one-tonne iron keel, has 156 buoyancy chambers and can carry 32 people. She's a bit of a local icon, these days. But by the time we got our hands on her, *Rescue III* was also a bit tired and beaten up. She was, to put it mildly, in need of some TLC. So that's what I did in the winter and spring of 2022. Stripped her right back, sanded her, took out a bit of rust and rot, patched her up and gave her a facelift, all with the aim of getting her looking as pretty as you can make a 70-year-old dame look.

It has been long, laborious, often strikingly repetitive work. It was dirty and dusty and I wouldn't recommend working with resin to anybody. But it was ultimately rewarding.

As you read these pages, you might see some parallels between me and *Rescue III*.

I'm not 12 tonnes, but I'm a big man, which is what gave me my natural advantages during my long rugby career. Some people might joke when they see me now that I turn about as quickly as a big old displacement hull. I'm a bit dinged up too, both mentally and physically. There have been plenty of times when, to put it mildly, I've needed TLC, too. It's been a full-time job for me, and just like with the boat, I couldn't have accomplished what I have without helpers.

I played 45 Tests as a tighthead prop for the All Blacks and can remember most of them pretty well. What I struggle to remember is what I did yesterday. Sometimes, at my most frustrated and frustrating, I'll start a sentence and forget what I was talking about halfway through.

At first, I wasn't sure why I had become like this. I had a load of questions piling up. Why was my mind wandering? Why did I find I needed to concentrate so hard on tasks that I used to be able to do without thinking?

Why was I plagued with crushing headaches? Why could I no longer relate to the players I was coaching? Rugby was what I knew best, so why didn't I know it anymore?

Why, after being referred to as a 'gentle giant' more times than I would like to count, was I not so gentle anymore? Why was I so thin-skinned these days? Why was I so quick to anger? Why was I hurting the ones closest to me, the people I loved? Why did I end up in the French judicial system, pleading guilty to the sort of offence that would bring shame upon me, one that I could never have imagined myself committing?

Why did I forget my son's name? Why did I keep thinking about dying? Yes, dying. And why did the prospect start to seem so appealing?

Why was alcohol the only thing that numbed the pain? Why was I so fucked up?

Like *Rescue III*, I was a vessel, sometimes empty, sometimes rudderless, adrift. Without urgent attention, I was in danger of sinking.

The questions crowding in on me were like a rising storm. But for too long, I didn't want to know the answers. I was a simple man, with simple pleasures. I still am, at heart. I had a rugby life and an away-from-rugby life, but for a while there, everything about my existence was impossibly complicated. But even with the walls closing in on me, I ignored it. I'm a Kiwi male. That's what we do.

I ignored it until one day, I couldn't ignore it any longer.

I needed answers.

I needed to find out if I was worth trying to fix.

I had to do something I've never felt comfortable doing. I had to ask for help.

When I started looking for answers, the information I was given wasn't always what I wanted to hear. I started hearing that my brain was damaged. Of course, I didn't want to believe it, but I saw the MRI scans and the bleeds that they revealed. I couldn't argue with those. And in light of them, a lot of what was happening to me began to make sense.

My prognosis, they said, was uncertain, because so much about the brain remains a mystery. I'm not the same person I was when I was younger. In five years' time it's highly likely I won't be the same person who wrote this book.

But I'm still Carl Hayman, and this is my story.

I

PAU, 2016–18, FALLING DOWN

ON THE NIGHT I assaulted my wife Natalie, I thought I had hit rock bottom. I thought that my life could not get any messier or debased. I thought that the distance between the person who I thought I was and the person I had become could not get any greater.

I was wrong on every count.

If there is a lesson I learned during my time in the little French town of Pau, it's that things can always get worse.

If I look back at it, the incidents in Pau were a manifestation of what had begun happening to me earlier in Toulon, but I didn't see it for what it was at the time. In fact, it wasn't until

I saw the scans of my brain that some of the things about me and my recent life that had baffled me began to fall into place.

Towards the end of my playing career, I began to have trouble with emotional regulation. I guess some people would look at that and say it's just a fancy way of saying you're having mood swings, and pretty much everyone has those at times in their life. But even at the time, I think I sensed there was more to it.

It wasn't just a matter of getting angry and irritable. At team meetings, I found myself welling up when talking — literally holding back tears. It's French rugby, you might say, a game played with a high emotional quotient, but I'm not even talking about stirring pre-match speeches. I'm talking about midweek meetings about the dry, technical aspects of the game.

I'd start choking up talking about stuff that didn't have any emotional significance whatsoever. I was so super-sensitive that I'd find myself short of breath and struggling to finish sentences. I now understand this to be the first real sign of cognitive decline, but I didn't recognise it as such because in other areas, I was fine. I wasn't having any issues with memory — nothing that gave me pause for thought, at any rate.

I finished my career in a blaze of glory, playing for Toulon. By the end of 2015, I was financially secure, and I was also entitled to live on le chômage. This is an important part of the French welfare system. It loosely translates as the dole, but it is slightly more complex than that. Here in New Zealand, there is a stigma attached to receiving the dole. In France, le chômage is intended to tide people over when they have recently left employment and have yet to find work. There's no stigma whatsoever: it is just baked into the French way of life. This income source gave me a bit of space to breathe after spending the bulk of the past two decades hammering myself in the world of professional rugby, without immediately dipping into the savings that I was planning to use to set my family up for life.

The first three months of retirement were great. I wasn't training and was putting on the kilos while enjoying my beers. The way I looked at it, I had worked bloody hard and it was time to relax for a bit. Charlie, my third child, was born around then. We owned our home in Carqueiranne, a village we loved. We were happy there. We'd made a real effort to integrate and speak the language. Natalie would go to the markets every Thursday and we'd adopted a husky called Vega. We were really settled.

But while it felt like a version of domestic bliss, I was always aware that it wasn't 'home'. We were planning our next move. Nat liked the idea of the kids going to a French school. I didn't mind the idea, but New Zealand — my real home — was starting to call pretty loudly, too. I had a loosely formed plan. We would return to New Zealand, find a farm and give the kids the kind of upbringing I'd had. I wouldn't necessarily do the hard yakker — the early mornings, the hard, physical labour: I'd get a manager on the place. But I would be back on the land where I felt I belonged. I couldn't imagine anything better, and I assumed Nat felt the same way.

At the end of 2015, we returned to New Zealand for Christmas and to enjoy part of the Kiwi summer. As soon as I was back, it really hit home — excuse the pun — how important it was for me to be back on the land and be close to my family again. I'd lined up a number of properties to have a look at, but I was struggling to get any direction or enthusiasm from Nat. She'd been in television before we shifted to France, and I wondered if it was a desire to get back into that industry that was making her reluctant to move to coastal Taranaki. I suggested she set up a meeting at TVNZ and I'd start looking for land in the Kumeū area, west of Auckland. Even that didn't seem to appeal to her. I assumed she'd lost a bit of confidence, having been out of the industry for a while. But that wasn't it. It turned out we had radically different ideas of what our future should look like.

I had stayed in professional rugby far longer than I had ever planned or expected to. It was the desire for financial security that drove me. When I brought down the curtain on my career, I took immense pride in the fact that I had literally played through pain to set up my family's future. I suppose I felt it entitled me to call the shots. I saw a return to the land as a reward for all that hard work. Nat didn't seem to see it that way, and I was bemused. I was presenting her with a lot of options, none of which she seemed very keen on.

She insisted she wanted to return to France and put the kids through school there. I could see the attraction for her and how a life experience like that could broaden the kids' minds. But I knew that if we returned, I'd have to get a job. If I'm totally honest, I resented that prospect. I couldn't think of anything that I could do that I would enjoy. Although I eventually caved and agreed that we would go back to France and give it a go, my mindset was negative right from the word go. It was the beginning of the end of our marriage.

I had heard that Simon Mannix, who had enjoyed a brief All Black career before playing and coaching in Europe, was looking for someone to coach the forwards at Pau, a little town in the shadow of the Pyrenees. The town itself wasn't much of a drawcard. If I had to describe it, I'd probably call it a kind of French version of Hamilton. But it was right in the foothills of the mountains: you didn't have to travel far for the kinds of recreational opportunities that I liked, and that was something. As for the job, I had no real interest in coaching. I didn't think it suited my personality. But I thought I could do a job for Pau and set my family up.

We rented the house in Carqueiranne out and moved to Pau. Mostly, I just felt like shit getting back on the rugby treadmill. That probably sounds odd to anyone who would kill to be involved with sport for a living. After all, I was back involved with the game that I still loved. But when you tell yourself that part of your life is finished and then you find yourself back immersed in it again, it can take you to a dark place mentally. Coaching isn't everyone's cup of tea. Coaching in France is a brutal workplace at the best of times and this wasn't the best of times. People talk about the values and spirit inherent in rugby but they don't mean a thing in coaching. It's utterly ruthless, because the owners don't share that spirit. There are a whole bunch of capable coaches competing for a limited amount of jobs. You can be summarily fired without warning. If you're not being fired, you're spending your time worrying if somebody else at the club is eyeing your job.

There are a number of great coaches in France who might dispute this, but it seems to me you have to be a politician first and a coach second to make it in that environment. It was a stumbling block for me because I never possessed the political smarts. Another aspect troubling me was that I never felt I had the necessary distance from the game to deal with the players in an appropriate way. I couldn't be one of the boys, but nor could I get comfortable dishing out orders and instructions to guys I had been playing with and against just a year or two before. It was too weird.

I had imposter syndrome, big time. There is a lot of video work in coaching — analysing video, producing video clips and presenting. As a player, I had appreciated coaches who could present sharp video analysis, like Wayne Smith, for example. The first time I fronted at my office, I didn't know how to operate a computer. Luckily, we had an Argentine guy on staff, Andrés Bordoy, a former Pumas front-rower, and he spent a lot of his time showing me the ropes. Still, in those early days in particular, most of my days were based around trying my hardest not to fuck up.

Yet even with all that angst and doubt, I felt I was doing an okay job on the training field. When. I joined, Pau was a relegation side. What I mean is that at the start of the season the principal goal of the team was to not get relegated from the Top 14. Everything we might achieve over and above that was a bonus. But in my first year as forwards coach, we nearly made the play-offs and I felt we were putting some good structures and systems into place. The feedback from Simon was good, and I trusted him enough to use him as a sounding board for the other stuff that was going on in my life. Because both of us knew something was amiss.

My physical exercise regime was good, so I was physically in good shape. But mentally and spiritually, I was a mess. As the season wore on, I should have been feeling more at home and comfortable with what I was doing. Instead, I would wake in the middle of the night and check my watch. If it was 2 am I'd let my head sink back on the pillow and feel a glow of contentment because it meant I had four more hours until I had to go to work. If sleep didn't come easily, I'd keep checking the watch to see that time ticking down. I had begun to dread going to work. Unlike playing, coaching is a lot more like a nine-to-five job, except it's a given that you're expected to work long hours. Players express their macho side by lifting bigger and bigger weights and hitting bags harder. Coaches show how tough they are by how many hours they work. In both cases it can be destructive.

The hours were a problem. But there was far more to it than that. When you step out of the playing environment, you suddenly realise how abnormal it is. I wouldn't say I ever craved the limelight or the glory that came with being a professional rugby player, but when I gave it up it still felt like a part of me had died. I didn't know who I was anymore. I used to be Carl Hayman, accomplished tighthead prop. Who was I now? Carl Hayman the coach? That didn't make sense to me, because it's never who I wanted to be.

I'd spent my professional life based on stats. What was I bench-pressing? What was I squatting? How many tackles did I make? How many lineouts did we lose? How many points do we need to make the play-offs? My inputs, my key performance indicators, were based on numbers. While rugby was my sole focus, it was all pretty simple. But either the numbers had disappeared or the calculations had become obscure. There was no readily available number that would tell me how effective I was as a communicator of my coaching ideas. Worse, there was nothing to measure how well I was doing as a husband or dad.

Something was broken. I would come home and tell Natalie that something was wrong with me, something that I couldn't fully explain or work out internally. She tried her best to help. She was big into nutrition and concentrated on making sure that I was eating well. But no matter how hard I tried to get a grip, to regulate my emotions, I just sank lower. When she asked me to help with the kids, I didn't embrace it. I chafed at it. I know it sounds selfish, but I just wanted to come home and try to forget about the world, not be swallowed up in more tasks. I would come home after a long day staring at a screen, more often than not with a splitting headache, and the last thing I wanted to do was a bunch of domestic chores. All I wanted to do was kick back and crack a beer.

That was one of the issues that neither of us tackled: my drinking. I didn't really consider myself to be a big drinker. Typically, I'd abstain during the week, and while I'd go out for beers after the game, it wasn't excessive. On Sunday, I'd normally drink while I did some jobs around the house and settled in to watch rugby on TV. There might have been the odd binge on a night out, but nothing that wasn't in line with how I'd drunk most of my playing career. I didn't think it was a problem. Nat saw it differently. She had been worried about it for some time, before we even shifted to Pau. After our marriage had ended, she told me that the real reason she had no desire to settle on a block of land in rural Taranaki was that she couldn't imagine living with me and my boozing in an isolated place.

Drinking had gone from being a recreation to serving as a crutch. I suppose I was self-medicating. I knew something was wrong with me and I was scared.

By now I'd started to notice that my cognitive abilities were deteriorating. The starkest example of this was when I was trying to arrange a passport for my son. I couldn't remember his name. I was on the phone to New Zealand, talking to a woman who was processing the details and there was this agonising gap of about 25 seconds where I was trying to open the right file in my brain that would give me access to this simple piece of information. It wouldn't come. In the end, I had to say to this poor, obviously bemused woman: 'I'm really sorry, I've forgotten. I've forgotten my son's name.' I got off the phone, embarrassed, agitated — and scared.

I've mentioned that coaching was largely a digital exercise. Athletes responded better to showing than telling, so a lot of our work away from the field was done on screens. But I couldn't go anywhere without my book. People probably thought I was just old-school, that it was quaint, but it was out of sheer necessity. If a player asked me something — even the simplest question — I needed to have the answers written down somewhere that I knew I could access easily. When I didn't have my book with me, I felt exposed. One day, a player asked me what the team was for the week. I had just emerged from a meeting of the coaching staff where we'd just settled the side — the most basic piece of coaching business: who plays. But standing there, I found I couldn't remember what we'd discussed literally five minutes earlier. I'd walked out of the meeting and lost that information immediately. I was frustrated, but I was also shaken. You can look at each of these episodes in isolation, and excuse them. The odd 'senior moment': who cares? We all have them from time to time, don't we?

But the excuses were wearing thin, and there were other things going on at the same time. Some of these worried me. Some of them should have worried me. I knew I shouldn't be suffering headaches in the way I did. They would greet me when I woke up and, at their worst, accompany me throughout the day. There was also the stuff I hoped I'd left behind in Toulon, but which had travelled with me to Pau: the inability to regulate my emotions, extreme sensitivity and irritability. There were also the weird feelings of déjà vu. I had begun to experience these towards the end of my playing days. I'd be on the field and I'd have this strange conviction that I'd done the exact same thing before, that I'd already played this match. Now, at Pau, it was happening more regularly. I was disoriented by it, but didn't think that much of it. Knowing what I know now, I ought to have seen it for what it was. Déjà vu can be a sign of stress and exhaustion, but there's also evidence that it can be a symptom of more serious neurological conditions.

At home, things were heading in the wrong direction with Natalie. It was painful then, and even now, I find it hard to talk about those days. We were growing apart. Every conversation seemed to start with good intentions but then descend into petty disagreements and a full-blown argument. And every single time I'd take stock and wonder how it had got to that point. 'I'm not an angry person,' I would think. 'Why am I getting like this?'

It all culminated one day when I took the kids out for a day by the Ousse River, just out of town. I took half a dozen beers with me and was drinking them while the kids played. It's my biggest regret. I had vowed never to put the kids in a position where they'd see me drinking and putting them in potentially unsafe positions. Nothing untoward happened during the day. I'm a big guy and six beers over the course of a day wasn't going to have a massive effect on my behaviour or sobriety, but that's not the point. It was dumb, irresponsible decision-making.

I got home and Nat was furious, absolutely livid. The short story is we had a massive fight. She tore into me — for good reason — and added a couple of reviews of my parenting skills I thought at the time crossed the line. It all got too much. I swiped at her with the back of my open hand. It connected. I never had any intention to cause physical harm, but on any analysis, it was a stupid, dreadful thing to do. I could load up the excuses — I had a shitty job, my marriage was crumbling and I was having a really bad day — but none of them stand up to any scrutiny. Plenty of people deal with shit like that and don't hit their wives, especially a wife who had no chance of defending herself against a six-foot-four former front-rower.

I was immediately flooded with guilt and shame and I thought, not for the first time: 'Fuck, I've hit an all-time low here.'

But just like the other times, I was wrong. I hadn't finished sliding yet.

Natalie kicked me out and locked the door. Instead of walking away I made some terrible choices. It was December, the pit of the French winter, and it was bloody cold. I decided that even if I was obviously not welcome in the marital bed, I needed to get inside, get in the spare room and warm up. By that stage, Nat had a friend with her and it was pretty obvious they weren't going to let me in. I made a fairly clumsy attempt to kick the door in. Things are pretty foggy at this point but I can only assume that I didn't try too hard because I'm not sure a door would be a match for me if I meant business. The police arrived. I knew one of the gendarmes: he had been down to training at Pau and had got to know me and the rest of the coaching staff. How, he asked, had I found myself in this kind of trouble? He knew me as a 'gentle giant'. I've heard that plenty of times in my life.

I was taken to the station and formally interviewed. It was some time before they told me Nat had indicated she didn't want to take it any further. I was thinking rationally enough to know that this wouldn't have been out of any feelings of charity towards me. She knew I'd be sacked from my role at the club and everybody would lose in that scenario. By the time I left the station, it seemed as though we were finished with police involvement.

I left the home and even if the marriage wasn't officially over at that point, I'd literally done the damage. I still find myself short of breath and have to catch myself when I think of the turmoil I put Nat and the kids through in those days.

But I hadn't finished falling. Over the next few months, I self-medicated with alcohol. I couldn't function at work. I was going in every day, spending the first part of each working day on the stationary bike, trying to sweat out the booze and make myself feel better about the person I was. I don't know how or why I was there, but I was trying and failing to do my job. Simon knew I was a passenger by this point. People, good people like Andrés, were covering for me and picking up my slack, but I didn't know why. I mean, my whole world had caved in because I was an idiot. Why would anyone care enough about me to try to save my job? Why didn't they hate me as much as I hated myself?

One of the toughest things I had to do was pick the kids up from my old home and drop them to school. Without fail, I'd drop them off and cry all the way to work. I might have been living in the same country and working in the same profession, but the glory days and success of Toulon, both on and off the field, seemed like they belonged to a different world, to a different life. I was pretty sure I didn't want the life that mine had been reduced to.

This might be hard to read for many people but I don't think my story is an honest one unless I tell you that this was when I decided to end my life. I'd chosen the method, the time, the place.

On those trips from the kids' school to work, I would compose the suicide note in my head. Each version started the same way: 'Sorry, your dad wasn't good enough...'

Suicide would be the one thing I could do properly.

Well, I'm alive to tell this tale. I can't fully explain why, but it probably comes down to this: I might have been filled with self-hate, but there were still people out there who cared enough about me to try to help. Like those at work covering my arse every day, like Andrés. Like Steffon Armitage and Jamie 'Whopper' Mackintosh, who took me in when I didn't have a home. For a while I'd alternate between their places.

Both Steffon and Whopper were good mates. Whopper knew my problems ran much deeper than a domestic breakdown and he was trying hard to get me through it. Perhaps the reason I stepped back off the ledge was as simple as thinking I couldn't be all bad if people like Whopper and Steff were willing to help me get my life back on track.

It made what was to come later even harder to comprehend.

I hated the thought of abusing Whopper and Steffon's hospitality, though, and wanted somewhere to bring the kids, so it led to another terrible decision.

I bought myself a little flat in Pau. It wasn't much to look at — a concrete-block thing — but it was right across the road from the supermarket. I came to know it as my 'Depression

Den'. I got into a destructive routine: leave work, visit the kids, feel terrible when they'd grab my leg and beg me not to go, leave them, arrive home, go to the supermarket, buy a bottle of spirits, return to my flat and use the alcohol as a Band-Aid. I didn't care what spirits I drank: it just had to be top shelf and strong enough to blot out the pain.

I knew I had a problem. I'd written a brutally difficult, confronting email to my family back in New Zealand in May 2017, addressing my drinking.

Hi Guys,

I need to be really honest with you all.

I have a drinking problem and have done for some time. Since I have finished rugby I have slowly started to lose control of my life.

Part of me turning my life around is admitting my problem and asking for help. With the drinking comes depression which I believe I'm also suffering.

I have a meeting with a counsellor tomorrow to try and get to the bottom of the problem. It's going to be a long road but it's something I need to do for myself and Nat and the kids. I'm really sorry and ashamed of what I have become.

I love you all loads. I'll try and touch base with you all over the next few days and have a chat.

Carl

Needless to say, although the email showed insight and self-awareness, my drinking problems didn't end with confronting them. Life trundled on in a destructive cycle of drinking, hangover, guilt, headaches and drinking until I mustered up what courage I had left and admitted to Simon that I was unwell and needed help. He went to the team doctor and they came up with a plan, which started by sending me to a rehabilitation centre in Orthez, about 20 minutes out of Pau on the road to Bayonne and Biarritz. I was a permanent resident for the first fortnight but then could check myself in and out during the day.

I kept an email diary of sorts, as much to keep my mind active as it was to let friends and family know how I was. Some of the spelling and grammar is pretty sketchy, so I've fixed some of the worst of the mistakes for ease of understanding. The diary isn't a bad indication of where my mind was: in other words, it's all over the show.

May 6, 2018:

Hi guys, just an update.

Day 1.

Jamie and Steff picked me up from the house and we travelled down to Orthez. Boys, thanks for the supply bag of goodies as the meals are small! I'll be playing on the wing in no time.

Arriving at the place was a bit like, what the fuck is this place? A massive château out of the Addams family and is possibly haunted! After the check-in formalities I was down to the accom wing to find my new digs. A bizarre experience having a lot of people talking and a few recognising who I was. This made me a little anxious but at the end of the day didn't bother me greatly as all the people here are in the same boat.

My first meeting with my doc was very positive and I am confident that before I leave here I will understand why I am like I am and develop a plan to ensure I can stay on track and be as productive as I can be in life.

The dynamics of the place are very interesting, almost in a prison type set-up (going off what I have watched on TV), you have fresh meat like me and the old hands who are here and about to leave and know the ins and outs of the place. Met two very nice people in Evonne and Ludo. Evonne has a hell of a story. Run out of Paris by the law a few years ago and been done for DIC twice in two days. Ludo the second is a fireman and loves training so we are off for a run this afternoon.

Horrible sleep first night here my bed is about 5 foot long and they have been giving me Valium. I felt like shit this morning and said I would préfère whiskey next time :-) as it was horrible. They know best so will just go with it.

I'm happy to be here and although the grounds are very small there is a 600 metre running track which I blasted around yesterday. And will continue to do so for the duration of my stay here. As my programme is not very intense, in my spare time here I'm going to ask to start work on the grounds as there is shit everywhere and there is an abandoned glass house which is overgrown so will offer to weed and fix it up so other patients here can spend some time there. I don't want to take on too much but I can't sit still for too long as you all know.

Leaving work has been hard, very sad to not be with the team as we are 4th now and I think we can really do great things but I know in the state I was in I was no use to them. I hope to come back stronger and make a real difference for the end of season.

I miss the kids loads but as of next week we can have visits and I'm allowed out to town in the afternoon (blow the bag on return) so I'll be looking forward to that.

I'll keep a daily diary and send through an update from time to time.

Love you all.

Carl

March 8, 2018:

Day 2.

Not much happening today. Took three other people to do some yoga and relaxation with them. I was the most qualified so ran a Fitness session for them. Nothing too much as I thought I might kill one of them.

After I had some lunch and ran 10 k round my 600m track. A bit sore tonight but just enjoyed doing something.

Had a bit of homework to do today so attacked that so I'm ready for the shrink when he opens up my head and finds mould, rust and probably some old car keys. Never mind. That's what we are here for.

Allowed out next week so am going to try to get the kids down. I think Steff is going to bring them down which will be great.

Bit of a shit dinner tonight so am into my goodie box. People are nice here they are all fucked up in their own special way which makes it a nice environment.

Not much else to report.

Day 3

Feeling shit today after a heavy night of Valium. I asked not to take it but they said because I'm not sleeping I need to take it. It is worse than a hangover.

Usual crew up to the gym for yoga and fitness. One lady is blind so she needs a bit of help but she said she is feeling a lot better in her back after two days of yoga so that was really positive. Finished up there and was back for a meeting with the doc. Talked to him about my drug intake and asked to cut it back please. Group work in the late morning talking about saying no and communications. Nothing too exciting there.

After lunch went for a run. 35 min and 5.5 k light today after yesterday's 10k. Was a bit bored after so swept all the smokers area of leaves and cleaned it up. Need a good smokers area eh Mum! Off to an AA meeting tonight with some other people here so should be fun.

Few issues around seeing the kids. I asked Nat if Jamie or Steff can bring the kids Wednesday so I can see them (their only afternoon off) but ... no they have sport and can't come so am trying to work something out. Not ideal as it's the one thing I was mostly looking forward to. I can only get out with 24 hours notice and for the afternoon. See how that progresses.

Everything going good, have set myself 3 goals here.

1 Define who I am.

2 What actions/words correspond with who I am.

3 what are my activities/projects am I doing that correspond to the above.

This should give me a good idea of where I want to go and direction when I leave.

After that planning my weeks and having time for what's most important is key. The rest is going in the bin.

Love to all,

Carl

March 10, 2018:

Day 4 Friday, Sat 5

I'm struggling today I need to see the kids. I'm feeling
sad and lonely. The drugs are having a bad effect on me.
I have asked a number of times to stop them completely
but they insist I need them. No yoga crew today so I went
for a walk with a lady I have become friends with here
called Evonne. Few laps around the compound and done.

Yesterday had a few exercises to do for my memory
to get my brain working again, not too successful for me
but I wasn't too worried.

About to watch the France England game so that
should be interesting.

I'm having some really strange feelings here and
almost scared of going back out or back to normality.
Here my life is simple. I think a huge factor when I go
out is going to be to strip back my life to the 'beer' lol
minimum, what's important. The rest can wait.

I have been thinking of a project to do once I get
out to give myself some focus and was talking with
my climbing friend Franck. We are looking at making
an ascent on Cho Oyu 8th largest mountain in the
world at 8200 odd metres (oct 2019). Early days yet
but I'm already training hard in my compound. I need
something to work towards and something like this
would be ideal.

I hope to see the kids soon. I miss them every day and am allowed out next week so will try and see them somehow. I think Whoppa and Steff will help us out there.

Off to watch the rugby. Steff and Whoppa go well tonight boys! All of us here and the rest of the region are behind you guys. Funny when you look from the outside in and everyone here talks about how well you guys are doing.

Love to all,

Carl

There were more emails and notes, but I think you get the picture. I was in a bad way. This was not where I ever envisaged Carl Hayman sitting: at a desk in a care facility for alcoholics and addicts, missing my kids, missing rugby, contemplating exactly who I was and what my future held. It seemed implausible, impossible even.

Once the course was over, I left the facility. But you remember what I said about things getting worse before they get better?

In about September or October of 2018, Nat indicated that she wanted full custody of the kids because she wanted to relocate to New Zealand. I can't properly articulate my emotions from back then, but it was a mixture of anger and confusion. That had been *my* plan. New Zealand was where I had wanted to be: on a farm with my family around me. Now I was stuck in a job I never wanted, living in a town I never wanted to live in, in a house that I associated with misery, while my kids were going home without me.

A short time later I was at the rugby club trying to climb back on the coaching horse when I got a call from the police. They wanted to have a chat with me. I told Simon I was just popping down to the station and would be back later. Instead, they questioned me about the night I hit Natalie again and next thing I knew I was in *garde de vue*, or police custody, spending the night in a cell with a bunch of random drunks, druggies and petty criminals. I must have asked myself the following question about 1000 times that night: 'What the fuck has just happened?'

The next day I was handcuffed, put in the back of a car and driven across town for a psychiatric evaluation. This was a complete mindwarp. I'm not taking away the severity of what I did to Nat, but there had been a lot of time between then and now and I was a completely broken, emotionally shrivelled man.

They were shooting a mouse with an elephant gun.

A court date was set for the following May but I was pretty paranoid by now. I couldn't see a happy ending. In my mind, everyone was out to get me.

Those feelings and the distrust I felt started to bleed into my work. Natalie had remained friends with many of the players' wives and rightly or wrongly, I got the sense they all hated me.

As a coach, it pays not to be too close to your players. If you fall out with them, it sours your working relationship. The way my life had panned out meant that I had broken that rule, and inevitably, I did fall out with my players. But it so happened that the two I fell out with most spectacularly were the ones I had leaned on so heavily in my darkest days.

My problem with Steff came about through really petty shit. He'd been working hard to fight his way back from a serious Achilles injury and had declared himself available for our away game at Racing. It was to be played on artificial turf and I just didn't think it was a great idea. I pushed back against him playing, wanting him to wait a week more. He unloaded on me, reminding me how he had been there for me but I wouldn't even back him up at the selection table. Steff and I had been mates since Toulon, quite apart from the kindness he'd shown me in my troubles. I loved the bloke, so this rocked me and reminded me why I never wanted to get into coaching in the first place.

My falling out with Whopper, who I had encouraged the club to sign, had far more damaging ramifications. Trouble had been brewing there for a while. One day he confronted me about something to do with Natalie and I told him to mind his own business. We maintained a fragile working relationship, but it all shattered on New Year's Eve. I had been to the gym at the club for a good training session with Craig Burden, a livewire South African hooker who was living with me between contracts. Once we had finished our workout, we started chatting about how it was New Year's and we should go to town. This was stupid decision number one, given I had not long ago completed a residency at Orthez for alcohol addiction.

We had a couple of beers — literally a couple — and headed into the Boulevard des Pyrenees, which is a street where most of the town's nightlife is, much like The Strip in Christchurch back in the day. The team was having a function at a bar so we headed that way, which was stupid decision number two. Needless to say, Natalie and I were not getting along, and I was anxious to avoid a confrontation. I believe I messaged Whopper saying I hoped she wasn't there. Stupid decision number three.

When Craig and I arrived, it was obvious Whopper had taken exception to my message. He grabbed me by the shirt and was aggressive. I should have left but there was a really toxic atmosphere and the confrontation was hard to avoid. We started wrestling and I caught my head on the edge of a railing, so there was a bit of blood.

It was crazy. I was a coach and I was in a confrontation with one of my players, one who had been a good mate, in a public place. Madness. We got out of there before it escalated further. Craig was blown away. He was like, 'What the fuck just happened?' It was hard to explain.

We went back to my place and next thing I knew Whopper and Steff were outside and Whopper was yelling: 'Let's finish this now.' I told him we'd sort it out in the morning, but he wouldn't leave and smashed the window of my front door. I ended up calling the cops. Nothing much happened, as far as I could tell, other than the fact that Whopper and Steff left.

The next morning, I called Simon Mannix straight away to tell him I'd messed up. Craig really wanted me to push the line that I was the innocent party and that he would back me up on that, but I knew better. I was the one who had a booze problem, who had recently done a stint in rehab, and even though I wasn't drunk that night, I'd put myself in a bad situation around alcohol again. There was nobody else to blame for that except myself. I knew how it was all going to play out. I didn't really care.

I met with Simon and he told me that three players had gone to the president to complain about me and, apparently, the way I had talked to another player's wife. That made me a little bit angry, but mostly just sad. It was a bit pathetic. I don't mind putting my hand up when I've screwed up and, as you can probably tell, I've screwed up a lot, but getting stitched up on some bullshit like that was tough to take.

The right thing happened, though. The players didn't want me there and I didn't want to be there. It was untenable, so I signed a severance deal. Simon, a guy I have a lot of time for, was great to deal with and he said the saddest thing from his point of view was that we — Whopper, Steff and I — were three guys who had done a lot for each other. He was right, of course. Those two had saved me from myself, in some respects, but the only way I could do anything for them in return was to save them from me, too. I had to leave.

At the time of writing, Steff is still playing, for Biarritz. I've been back in touch with him. I've thought about Whopper a bit over the past couple of years and have considered giving him a call. I'm never sure how I'd start the conversation. Maybe it would be something as simple as: 'Thanks for helping me leave professional rugby. It was long overdue.'

Because that is how I feel. It was an ugly way to end, but my first thought when I signed those severance papers was: 'Thank fuck for that.'

What a climb-down, right?

It wasn't that long ago that I was Carl Hayman, former All Black, professional rugby player, living the perfect life with the perfect family. It seemed like I'd reached the peak of a mountain I'd been climbing my whole life. But the person who was standing on that summit was a hollowed-out version of me. I didn't have to look much further back to find another version of myself: just a kid with a big body in a small town.

Where the hell did he go?

2

OAONUI, 1979–92, GROWING UP

STATE HIGHWAY 45, the Surf Highway, or just plain old South Road, leaves New Plymouth at the western end of town, near where I live now, and hugs the coast as it takes a wide berth from the maunga — the mountain — that gives the province its name, Taranaki.

The road has taken on a character of its own in recent years, with the tributaries that branch off it leading to some of the best surf spots in the country and, if you talk to the locals for long enough, the world. Some of the breaks take their names from the narrow roads that service them, like Ahu Ahu, Arawhata and Stent Road, while other spots have more exotic and sometimes ominous names, like Kumera Patch, Greenmeadows, Rocky Rights and Graveyards.

The Surf Highway carves its way through a number of towns — although it's taking bit of civic licence to call glorified crossroads 'towns'. There's Ōakura, Ōkato, Pungarehu, home to the Barrett clan, Rahotu, Oaonui and Ōpunake, before the road bends with the South Taranaki Bight and bisects the towns of Pīhama, Kaupokonui and Manaia. Finally, it reaches Hāwera, the largest urban area in South Taranaki, where 45 links back with State Highway 3 and heads down country to Whanganui and places beyond.

It is dairy country. The cow-to-human ratio tips heavily towards bovine. The fertile land of the Taranaki ringplain and the abundance of wet stuff from the sky make for perfect grass-growing conditions. To the outsider, it can appear to be a bit bleak and inhospitable, especially when dark clouds shroud the mountain and the wind, which finds little resistance as it shreds across the paddocks, whips off the Tasman Sea. To locals like me, however, who never get sick of being within arm's reach of the mountain and the sea, it's a place of real beauty whatever the weather.

Once it's your home it's always your home and they reckon that mountain acts like a giant magnet, pulling you back. I wouldn't disagree.

About the only relief from the grass and the cows and the utes is the oil and gas infrastructure. Stand on the old family farm on a clear day and when you look directly out to sea, past the beacon at the end of the property that warns ships that land is close, you can see Maui Platform A. The gas and condensate from the field comes ashore at Oaonui, where it is processed before being piped north to Methanex's methanol plants near Waitara and up country to the pipeline's terminus at the Huntly Power Station.

This is where I grew up, in the land of milk and gas.

My world pretty much extended from Kina Rd, Oaonui, where my parents Dave and Anne were sharemilkers — that is, they owned the herd they milked, but leased the land — past the family farm at 4745 South Road, and into Ōpunake, where I started school at St Joseph's and played sport, summer and winter, as often as I could.

I was the first child, born as spring was slowly turning to summer on November 14, 1979, at Ōpunake Maternity Hospital. Like many other small-town public services, the hospital was closed in the 1980s and the building was later saved and turned into a rest home. I'm pleased I have Ōpunake on my birth certificate rather than Hāwera or New Plymouth: it more accurately reflects where I come from. I'm in good company. Peter Snell, the three-time Olympic track gold medallist was born there, as were other luminaries such as former Prime Minister Jim Bolger, the brilliant All Black captain and flanker Graham Mourie — an almost mythical local figure in my youth — and pioneering Māori writer Jacquie Sturm.

Mum's family, the O'Rorkes, are a multi-generational Ōpunake family. Irish Catholics. These kinds of identifiers matter in rural Taranaki. They say you have to be careful about what you say and who you say it to around the coast because there's a good chance they'll be related to the subject of your ire.

Dad was a blow-in from Taihape. He came to Ōpunake to take over the butchery. Mum was a trainee hairdresser. I don't exactly know how they met but there's a high chance it involved one of the two pubs in town, the Club Hotel or the Ōpunake Hotel. They were a young couple. Mum was 18 when she had me and I suspect my impending arrival might have instigated the marriage. Sisters Stacey and Rebecca would come later.

My first years were spent as a 'townie', but I was still pretty small when Mum and Dad went sharemilking on a family property at Lower Kina Road. I travelled the 10 kilometres into Ōpunake every day to attend St Joseph's: the pull of the church ran strong in mum's family. But with about 18 months to go, I was taken out of St Joe's and went to Oaonui, which was a great little place — two classrooms and a roll of about 35 kids. Unfortunately, like the hospital, the school is no longer operational. The buildings still stand, but they're empty and the pool (with a giant crab painted on the bottom to try to discourage kids from diving in) is also empty, and unloved.

The dairy factory, Egmont, also went long ago as the industry moved to co-operatives. It had been a big local employer. I still remember reading the mournful 'Rest In

Peace' graffiti on the stainless-steel tank on the side of the building. The talk around town at the time was pretty bleak. The closure was seen as a big blow to the community. In 1989, Egmont Dairy merged with Moa Nui, with the milk going to Inglewood, before Moa Nui was folded into Hāwera-based Kiwi Co-op in 1992. Eventually, in 2001, Fonterra swallowed everything.

You can debate the economic pros and cons of consolidation as much as you like, but for many places, losing their factory meant losing a large part, sometimes all, of their identity. If you look at a map of Taranaki, there are a bunch of placenames that still feature, though they aren't really places at all anymore. Where there once would have been a hall, a school and a small dairy factory, now some of them don't even have a hall, let alone a school. It's such a shame how those staples of country life are being eliminated. The school was the centre of the community, with working bees and gala days connecting families that were otherwise spread far and wide.

Progress always comes at a cost.

For me, the loss of the factory meant the end of the odd rides I'd get down Kina Road with the Egmont tanker drivers we got to know. We had the first shed on the road, so I'd jump in when they took our milk and get dropped off when we'd finished collecting the rest.

I loved growing up on a farm. I can't imagine a better place to be a kid. You had space — literally — to grow and developed a type of self-reliance that is hard to replicate in an urban environment. You couldn't just pop down the road for entertainment or to grab McDonald's. You made your own fun, and often enough, your own food. If you woke up in the morning and were hungry, you made yourself something to eat because the chances were that mum and dad were down at the milking shed. If things broke, you fixed them. That tendency to rely on yourself can also have consequences. It's well documented that there are high rates of mental health issues amongst farmers: part of it is the sense of isolation, but the belief that you can fix everything yourself, even if it's your mind, has even more to answer for. I'd end up learning that lesson the hard way.

I loved farm machinery, so Grandad's place was heaven. He had a fleet of Massey Ferguson tractors. He had a 35, a little 135, a 165 and he ended up buying a 375, which was a four-wheel-drive tractor. He drew the line at buying a cab tractor: he was a bit old-school like that. In later years, my uncle, his youngest son, who's only a few years older than me, got into farm contracting and bought himself the latest John Deere cab tractor, which went against everything Grandad believed in, namely that sitting out in the open on a good solid bit of English iron was the only proper way to farm. But he hopped in the John Deere one day and went: 'Ooh. This is actually all right, isn't it?' He was in his seventies by then and it was too late to change his views on cabs or tractor brands, but I think there was part of him that might have started wondering if he'd been a bit stubborn all those years.

The tractors were put to good use during haymaking season, a big part of the rural annual calendar. All the neighbours would come together to help each other with their harvest. You'd go from farm to farm, everyone pitching in to help. It was long, hot work and always finished with everyone sitting down with quart bottles of beer in hand and admiring the shed stuffed full of square bales. Nowadays, with technology, haymaking is far less manual labour. It's pretty much all machine-driven. And instead of storing baled hay in sheds, it's shrink-wrapped and left in the fields. Haymaking as a red-letter day on the rural calendar has gone the way of small dairy companies and country schools.

As I got older, I developed an appreciation for the hours farmers put in. It was a good life, but it was a lot of hard work. Nevertheless, it was pretty much all I imagined myself doing. In a way my life seemed pretty prescribed from a young age, and I didn't mind that. Go to school, maybe do an agricultural sciences degree and then spend the rest of my life on the land with a family and a herd. The prospect appealed to me.

I guess rugby mucked up a good plan.

My early memories of footy mostly revolve around watching the Ōpunake seniors. The smell of liniment coming from the changing rooms, wandering around the field with half an eye on the game, half an eye on the caravan making hot chips. I liked climbing the macrocarpa trees that lined the Rec at one end and listening to the thuds of the tackles and the corresponding 'oohs' from the crowd. Later, when I got a bit older, I would get to operate the scoreboard and would be paid for my labours with a mince pie. Bliss.

The seniors wore Irish green jerseys, in keeping with the local Catholic affiliations, and while they didn't win championships, they had some good, tough players like the Flemings, Hank Schrader and Kevin 'Smiley' Barrett, who might be more famous for who he is father to these days, but was also a bloody good player himself, at his best as a raw-boned blindside flanker.

There used to be one club, sometimes more, for every small town in Taranaki. But club rugby in Taranaki, and elsewhere in New Zealand, has gone the way of dairy companies, and many old, proud identities have disappeared in round after round of mergers. Hāwera used to have two clubs — Athletic and the eponymous Hāwera — but those clubs merged with Waimate, from nearby Manaia, to form Southern. Eltham and Stratford were bitter rivals who have now combined, while Ōpunake, Rahotu and Ōkato all merged to form Coastal. It's always sad to see clubs disappear, but Coastal hasn't just survived as a club: it's thrived. That sense of community around the rugby team has remained, even if it represents a much larger footprint now.

Playing sport was a huge part of my childhood, too. Not just rugby. I was keen on basketball, touch rugby and cricket in summer. An aunt took me down to Ōpunake Rugby Club as a kid. That's where it all started, aged five. I wasn't that physically imposing back then, but it didn't take long. From the age of eight, I started to dwarf other kids. The size came with some drawbacks, though. My Grandad told me I needed a new gearbox because my body had outgrown my ability to move it around at any pace.

With playing and watching sport, Ōpunake Rec was the centre of my world. It's changed a bit over the years, with grandstands being demolished and rebuilt and the community sports centre on site being upgraded, but anyone who grew up in rural or small-town New Zealand will recognise the set-up: a couple of rugby fields in winter, a cricket oval in summer, clubrooms dominated by the bar and a bunch of team photos staring proudly out at you from the walls. Mourie's jerseys, that he collected from opponents around the world, also took pride of place on the wall.

The whole place was a focal point for the community, too. Saturdays were spent on the sidelines, then back to the clubrooms afterwards for beers. I'd hate to think what the drink-driving ratio was back then, but I'm pretty sure the cops would have been kept busy if they chose to focus on it. Truth be told, they were probably amongst the crowd at the bar as often as they could be.

Cricket was probably my first and most serious sporting love. I made the South Taranaki reps. This team would play

North Taranaki every year and go to the Riverbend Camp Tournament in Hawke's Bay, a highlight of the cricket summer.

I was reasonably handy. I fancied myself as a hard-hitting all-rounder. I'd bat at number 6 and bowl whenever I got a chance, though I probably lacked the yard or two of pace that I'd have needed to be really effective. I batted right-handed and bowled and threw with my left. I really enjoyed cricket as a kid. More than rugby. I'd listen to it on the radio out on the farm and probably had more dreams of making it as a cricketer than I did as a footy player, though that was another plan that rugby — and my physique — mucked up.

Although Dad helped out in coaching in both cricket — he was awarded loudest snorer at one of those Riverbend camps — and rugby, his passion was for the winter code. He'd played, not to any great level, but he loved the game and was one of the few players you'll hear about who transitioned from the midfield to the front row as farm nutrition began to take effect.

I wouldn't necessarily say his passion rubbed off on me, but all kids want to make their dads happy, and if watching me play rugby spun his wheels then I was more than happy to oblige. Food was definitely a big part of my early life. The freezer was always full and like many farmers' wives, Mum saw a big part of her role was to make sure her human livestock were well-fed. Christmases were epic, with cousins — both Mum and Dad were from large families — aunts and uncles all gorging themselves from a seemingly endless supply of meats, salads and puddings. The leftovers could last close to a couple of weeks, but as I got older and bigger, we'd streamlined the operation so that the scraps ran out shortly after New Year's Day.

While I spent more time with my maternal grandparents, Dad's folks had retired and moved from Taihape to Waverley, about halfway between Hāwera and Whanganui. I'd spend school holidays there and remember my Grandmother June being a big whitebaiter. June would make us a bunch of sandwiches and we'd jump in the family Mitsubishi Lancer and head to the Waitōtara River to try to get a catch for a feed of fritters.

When I think about it, I've spent a lot of my time catching stuff and eating it.

Once I left primary school, I went to New Plymouth Boys' High School (NPBHS) for my first year of college. I boarded in Carrington House, which has since been torn down — not before time, as it had more than a touch of Communist-era Bulgaria about its aesthetics and level of comfort.

The 1st XV in the year before I got to Boys' High had won the World championships. That team had Michael Collins, Brooke Wolfe, Reuben Thorne, Campbell Feather — now *that* was a really good team, so rugby was on a high at the school. I can't claim to have contributed to its success. I played, but even then, I was showing no talent. I think my team was C2 Gold. It was essentially the leftovers.

I hated boarding to start with. It turned out I was a homebody. It sounds funny to think of it in this way, but even at that age, 13, I reckon I could have run the farm for Dad. I knew how it worked, knew how to milk and if it was legal and had been an option at that point of my life, I would have chosen to leave school and be a farmer.

It might have been easier if I'd had a few mates in the hostel, but as a Catholic, I was a bit of a square peg in a round hole. Even as a boarder in third form (Year 9, these days), I'd get the blazer and tie on and head off to St Joseph's church in New Plymouth every Sunday for Mass. That was probably my last year of consistent worship as I became more and more secular in outlook. The Catholic kids in the area tended to go to Francis Douglas Memorial College, which also had a boarding house. I can't tell you why I didn't follow that path. It would have made sense, given Mum was raised in the church and that I was an altar boy. If you go into St Joseph's now, you'll still find an altar boy's cloak with my name on it. Perhaps it was because Dad was lukewarm about religion at best. The only time he went to church was at Christmas. I don't think he was too keen on its traditions or teaching and that might be why I ended up at both Oaonui Primary and NPBHS.

I got Dad into trouble during one of his rare trips to Mass. I must have seen him loading the car up with flagons to fill at the Club Hotel after church. In one of those quiet moments in the middle of the service when you're bored and just want to interact with your parents, I leaned across the pew and said a little bit too loudly: 'Hey, Dad. Didn't you want to leave early so we could go and fill those flagons up?'

It was pretty common for third formers to arrive in a new environment and be a bit overwhelmed. Especially at a big school like NPBHS, there are a whole lot of traditions and a hierarchy that you have to quickly get used to. Many of the boarders, like me, come from small towns or farming communities and a school like NPBHS, with about 1200 kids, can seem impossibly loud and chaotic. I'm sure it's a bit easier these days where much more attention is paid to the mental wellbeing of students, but if you get off on the wrong foot at a hostel, it is very easy to sink without a trace.

I liked school, but at that age, it took a while to adjust. I was homesick. There was a payphone by the bell tower and I'm not sure how many collect calls I made to Mum in those early days, telling her I was coming home.

Even in the third form though, I could see the immense pride the boys took in playing for the 1st XV, when the whole school would be let out early to line the terraces of the Gully Ground and cheer the team on in traditional matches against the likes of Auckland Grammar, St Patrick's College Silverstream, Hamilton Boys' High School and others.

As third-form boarders, we had our own version of the inter-school game. Every year, Niger House — a combination of our hostels — would take on Palmerston North Boys' High

School's College House. Niger House v College House was a big deal. Every morning, those in the team would wake early to go for a run before ending back at the Gully Ground for some more fitness drills. It was really beneficial for me at that age. For the first time, I began to understand what being fit meant. I could actually feel the difference. Before then, at the start of each rugby season I might run down Kina Road to my neighbour's gate and back, maybe do that two or three times, and call that pre-season training.

I'd made the team as a lock, and could play No. 8 at a pinch. We lost to College House. They had a kid called Grant Webb who would end up playing for Otago and end his career in Wales with the Newport Gwent Dragons. He was pretty handy at No. 8 and proved to be the difference between the two teams.

I'm not sure if something was stirring in me then. It probably wasn't, because I still had no discernible talent that elevated me above others. And even if it was, a far greater upheaval was to occur in my life beyond being sent to boarding school. In early 1993, my parents announced that the family was moving to Otago.

3

LONDON, 2020, DIAGNOSIS

IN JUNE 2019, I was at the wedding of a former Newcastle teammate, Ollie Phillips. It would end up being a life-changing day, not just for Ollie, one of the great characters in rugby and a really high-achieving guy, but for me, too.

It was here I became reacquainted with Alix Popham. The funny thing is, I can't really recall it, but he can, so it obviously happened. I'd played against Alix a couple of times: for the All Blacks against Wales and almost certainly when he was at Brive and I at Toulon. Alix is a force of nature. Ollie's wedding must have been around the time of his own diagnosis for early-onset dementia and probable chronic traumatic encephalopathy

(CTE). Rather than letting that news stop him in his tracks, Alix is going harder and faster at everything in life. He's started a lobby group, Progressive Rugby, aimed at making the sport safer, and he and his wife Mel have launched a foundation, Head For Change, to provide support to athletes, and families of athletes, who are living with early-onset dementia, chronic traumatic encephalopathy, or other degenerative brain diseases.

When his diagnosis became public at the same time as World Cup-winning England hooker Steve Thompson's, I flicked him a message of support. Who knew it would soon be the other way around.

Alix reached out to me at a point when I was near my lowest. I was struggling to get any tangible support in New Zealand. I was beginning to feel the sort of rage you feel when you're impotent against the system. I wanted the Accident Compensation Corporation to recognise that the problems I was facing on a daily basis were due to my profession, to the sport I played and loved, but I just kept hearing that I was depressed because I was going through a bad divorce and once I was clear of all that, I'd bounce back and be fine.

Try living inside my head and then see how that assessment looks. I know from first-hand experience what depression is. I know I'm not immune to it, but I also knew that this was different. It was agonising headaches, it was extreme sensitivity to light, it was the inability to construct simple sentences, it was the feeling that you've just lost a few minutes and have no idea where they went or what you were doing. That awful feeling when you find yourself driving purposefully in the car and have no idea where you're going. Weird stuff that was happening towards the end of my playing career, such as faulty emotional regulation, had spilled into my ill-fated coaching career at Pau and more troublingly, into my post-rugby life. This idea I clung to that all my problems would ease once rugby was in the rearview wasn't working out. I kept getting overly emotional even having the most basic conversations. Any criticism, implied or often just imagined, would send me into a world of hate.

I might well have been depressed, but it was because my head was broken and I couldn't articulate that fact to the people who, to some degree, could determine a big part of my future wellbeing with a few strokes of their pen. Having my claim rejected meant I couldn't get access to specialist post-concussion and neurological help. But in the end, it was the sheer arrogance and dismissive nature of the assessment that sent me into a downward spiral.

The more I thought about it, the more I wondered if I was truly going mad. If you think you're going mad, your natural reaction is to run as far from the issue as possible. Hunker down, try to shield yourself with a cloak of invisibility, or maybe a cloak of invincibility. Pretend everything is okay. It's just a passing phase. As soon as I get some time to relax, all this shit will stop.

That was what I'd done for close to a year. I was in a new relationship, but here I was, slowly but surely disintegrating at a time when I had a newborn daughter who had her own health issues, and a business I wanted to make the best of.

In the background, my partner Kiko, an English woman I had met on a charity bike ride for the late Doddie Weir's foundation, had been talking to Ollie, who was concerned for me and wanted to know if he could reach out to Alix. So I took a call. The unmistakably Welsh sing-song tones came down the line. 'Hello, Carl. I hear through the rugby grapevine you're having a tough time. I think I can help...'

That's what I needed to hear. Alix outlined what he and a few others were doing in terms of taking World Rugby to court. He explained the motivation. How players of our generation had an obligation not to allow the next generation to end up like we did. That appealed to me. A cry for help can sound quite selfish, but there was a much bigger issue at play here. He told me how many subconcussive hits he thought he had absorbed during his career, and it was a frightening number — not least because I had played a hell of a lot more professional rugby than Alix.

Most of all, I realised I wasn't alone. There is comfort in numbers: don't let anybody tell you different. He said he had talked to scores of rugby players in the same position as me, some still playing and some much worse off than me. Ex-players who were literally on suicide watch. The messaging to them from medical professionals had been similar: 'This thing with your head, it's depression. We can put you on antidepressants, blah, blah, blah...'

Alix outlined the case they were making and the testing procedure and encouraged me to think hard about submitting myself to it. Kiko and I were returning to the United Kingdom to visit her family, so there was an opportunity to kill two birds with one stone. Yet one thing was still holding me back.

It was this: fear. The fear of knowing can be worse than the fear of the unknown. I'd read and seen a lot of the material around the NFL and chronic traumatic encephalopathy. It wasn't curable, so perhaps it was better not to know.

I um'd and ah'd for a long time. Went back and forth in my own mind. I had lots of conversations with Kiko about it. We had a young daughter, Genevieve Ocean (Osh, long O like the O in Ocean, for short). What would it mean if I was really sick? Sometimes it felt as though that was all we talked about. Did I really want to find out if something was wrong with me? Or did I just want to get on with life, try to be the best dad I could and hope for the best?

We flew to the UK, and stayed with Kiko's family in Herefordshire near the Welsh border. I was so close to where Alix was based that I'd have been mad not to take advantage of the proximity. So I arranged to meet him. He talked me through his own fears and convinced me it was better to know, even if the diagnosis wasn't what you wanted to hear.

He told me how strange his emotions were when he found out he had early-onset dementia: how it was a relief. He talked about how his diagnosis had freed him. At last, there was something tangible about his disease. He didn't have to worry that his issues were imaginary problems. It allowed him to make plans. He knew what he was dealing with so could organise his present and his future accordingly. He's a bit different from me, a glass half full guy, but reaching the same place as Alix had done sounded a lot more attractive than the purgatory I was living through, so I agreed to go to London and have the testing.

As soon as we got to London, it occurred to me how much I needed help. I have travelled around the world and have been to London several times. I have efficiently and effectively used some fairly complex public transport systems in countries where a different language is spoken. Perhaps it was the anxiety about what I was about to undertake, but if it wasn't for Kiko, who herself had brain surgery and intensive care treatment at King's College Hospital in Camberwell, I would never have made it there. The London Underground was a bridge too far in my panic-stricken state, but Kiko somehow got me to my appointment on time.

The testing was gruelling. There are three rounds. You speak to a neurologist at the beginning for about an hour and a half. Then you undergo very thorough neuropsychological testing, which takes three to four hours. Finally you have a series of MRI (magnetic resonance imaging) scans.

I surprised myself at how well I did on some of the tests, but on others, I felt embarrassed. There was one test for memory where they read you out a short story and you had to recall as many details as possible. It wasn't a complex story but at the end of it I drew a nearly complete blank. The only thing I could utter was: 'It was a story about two lions.'

That, as you can imagine, was a deflating experience.

From there, it was a process of waiting for the results. When they came, it was confusing trying to sift through what was important and what wasn't. The MRI scans had been done with anisotropic diffusion technology (DTI, or diffusion tensor imaging), a step up from the standard tech, which can estimate the level of axonal (white matter) organisation of the brain.

The scans showed two distinct lesions in the cerebellum, but the radiology results were otherwise specified as unremarkable, which Kiko and I obviously took as good news.

Given I found some of the recall exercises close to impossible, while in other tasks I felt much more adept, I wasn't surprised that my neuropsychology report summary was mixed. Here are the key takeaways.

Focal cognitive testing revealed impairments in memory (both verbal and visual). Whilst he did benefit from information being repeated, he struggled to encode and retain information provided once. On the whole, performance on executive tasks was at the level expected, apart from on a task that fell in the Borderline Impaired range where he was required to deal with cognitive interference (Stroop). Immediate attention (Digit Span) as well as Semantic fluency (Animals) was mildly reduced, in the Low Average range and Processing Speed Index from the WAIS-IV was moderately below the level expected, in the Borderline Impaired range.

The summary concluded that I was suffering from moderate cognitive dysfunction affecting 'fronto-temporal regions in the main' but also with subcortical involvement.

Importantly, the report noted: 'Given the specific nature of the findings, it is unlikely to be as a result of mild to moderate levels of psychological distress... In my view these findings warrant further medical investigations given his relatively young age, history of multiple sport related head injuries and concussions, as well as issues with memory in day-to-day life.'

There was a bit to unpack there. There was even more when I received my diagnosis from Dr Steven Allder, the consultant neurologist.

With respect to Mr Hayman in particular, it is now possible to integrate all of this updated information and say the following things:

Firstly, Mr Hayman has been involved in sport in which there is a recognised high risk of suffering concussion and sub-concussive hits (both during training and in matches).

Making a diagnosis of Chronic Traumatic Encephalopathy (CTE) in Mr Hayman, given that he is still alive, means it is necessary to consider his clinical presentation compared to the most recent consensus document; this suggests that he has got the precise clinical profile that is a key requirement for considering this diagnosis.

Mr Hayman has got a high risk dosage of contact sports, with approximately 17 years as a professional rugby player. In addition, he is presenting with typical neuro-behavioural symptoms (for example, he is more short-tempered). Importantly, these symptoms are currently less marked than his cognitive symptoms.

Finally, Mr Hayman has a progressive presentation which is now causing a degree of functional impairment.

In Mr Hayman's presentation, there are no genuine clinical pointers to any alternative diagnosis. In my opinion, any additional investigations are unlikely to materially assist. However, of course, I have no objection to Mr Hayman undergoing further investigation to exclude the possibility of an alternative diagnosis.

In conclusion, while this is clearly a new entity, Mr Hayman's clinical picture is strongly suggestive of this diagnosis. Mr Hayman has been informed of my formulation. He has been encouraged to see his GP to seek further advice and support.

On the basis of the clinical assessment and information available to me at present, I consider that Mr Hayman does have evidence of brain injury from his involvement in contact sports. He has suffered multiple concussions and is now exhibiting progressive clinical symptoms consistent with a form of pre-senile dementia, and the precise diagnosis is mild Chronic Traumatic Encephalopathy (CTE). As a consequence of this, he does have all of those clinical symptoms that are consistently present; although they are at a mild level at this point my clinical experience suggests that they will, unfortunately, get worse. In addition, the functional impairment associated with Mr Hayman's symptoms is already having a significant impact on his ability to undertake his normal job.

By definition, as outlined above, mild Chronic Traumatic Encephalopathy (CTE) is a form of brain injury and it is resulting in permanent symptoms.

The recommendation was, simply, to undergo more testing in 12 months' time to see what regression had taken place in my existing symptoms and what, if any, new symptoms were presenting.

Alix had talked of the relief he felt at finally having the answers to his problems when he received his diagnosis. I wasn't quite there yet. I was more in a state of confusion. I mean, my scans were not perfect, not by any stretch, but they weren't *that* bad, were they? My psych testing fell below normal in some areas, but not in others. Yet here I was contemplating the news that I was definitely permanently damaged and it was only going to get worse. Even if I suspected this was the case beforehand, it was a lot to take in. Relief? Nah, that's probably not the word I would have been searching for immediately.

Kiko and I started asking questions and it slowly started to make sense. When you have disparate people working on separate parts of the process, they're working with limited information. The radiographers, for example, don't know they're looking at a former rugby player. They're looking at the brain with a view to finding more acute damage, like tumours or extraordinary changes or disintegration in the white matter.

It was the consultant neurologist who pulled all the pieces together to view the full picture. He could see the lesions, the cognitive decline and the sociability symptoms I was exhibiting and, along with my history, made the devastating diagnosis. It didn't stop Kiko and I searching for more answers. We wanted to reconcile the scans with the diagnosis. Unfortunately, the news didn't get a whole lot better. Two separate neurologists said they wouldn't expect to see some of the deterioration on my brain in a 70-year-old.

I don't have a great recollection of this time. If you asked Kiko, she would tell you the testing left me completely 'zonked'. She reckons I went rapidly downhill after the diagnosis, becoming depressed and anxious in equal measures. She recalls me telling her that the last eight or so years of my career had been played with the sole aim of setting up my family and now everything had broken down and my brain was wrecked. I told her that my life had been a complete failure.

Where others have taken their diagnosis as a signal to attack life and make the best of it, my inclination was to shrink from it. My confidence was knocked.

I eventually made the choice to join the lawsuit against World Rugby and the Rugby Football Union (England's governing body), and I'd later join the action against the French Rugby Federation. I also decided to go public with my diagnosis.

I told my story, which broke simultaneously on *The Spinoff* website and *The Bounce* newsletter, although almost immediately the story was picked up by all the major news outlets in New Zealand and many others around the world.

The first three paragraphs of the story were unflinching:

Carl Hayman was once estimated to be the highest-paid player in rugby. Now, less than six years after the end of his playing days, he has spoken of the disorientation he felt as his career was winding down, and the ceaseless headaches that plagued him and sent him into a spiral of alcohol abuse and frequent suicidal thoughts, culminating in a suspended prison sentence in France after admitting to charges of domestic violence.

'I spent several years thinking I was going crazy. At one stage that's genuinely what I thought. It was the constant headaches and all these things going on that I couldn't understand,' Hayman says.

The 41-year-old, once regarded as the finest tighthead prop in the world, now has an explanation. He received a shocking diagnosis after extensive testing in England that included a brain scan that can identify changes in the brain's white matter. He has been diagnosed with early-onset dementia and probable chronic traumatic encephalopathy, or CTE. It's a progressive brain condition which has been strongly associated with former NFL players and boxers. The 'probable' refers to the fact that it can only be properly diagnosed post mortem.

There was a really problematic line in that story. It was the first time I had been forced to confront the 'D' word. It might sound implausible, but after all the testing, and perhaps because I'd heard so much about what was happening in the US around the NFL, I was almost hyper-focused on the term

CTE. Again, this could come across as naïve, but the term early-onset dementia had never really entered my thinking. To see it sitting there in black and white gave me a huge shock. I rang the lawyer in the United Kingdom, who had also spoken to the reporter for the story.

'Is this true?' I asked.

It was. It was in the neurologist's report, but my eyes had skated over those words (which now appeared to me as though they were in bold type) and gone straight to CTE:

He has suffered multiple concussions and is now exhibiting progressive clinical symptoms consistent with a form of **pre-senile dementia**, and the precise diagnosis is mild Chronic Traumatic Encephalopathy (CTE).

I learned that day that CTE is a form of dementia. I knew people with dementia. I knew this was not a good outcome. The irony was that I was on this journey of discovery about my condition just as it became harder and harder to process new information.

My phone went mad that morning. A lot of it was messages of love and support, which was hugely gratifying but also overwhelming. The whole reason I had done the story so comprehensively was to tell it once and not have to tell it again, but the media were doing their job and following up on the story. I couldn't deal with the attention, so I jumped in the truck, headed down the coast and went and sat on my tractor for the day, occasionally checking my phone to see how many calls and messages I had missed. That left Kiko to deal with any media inquiries that came through the business phone — given there was a story written when we bought the Chaddy's Charters business, we weren't hard to find — and she put her maternal hat on, protecting a child — me — from the outside world.

If it was just the diagnosis and all the depression and anxiety that came with it, I might have coped. But life had another couple of curve balls to throw at me.

My mum had been diagnosed with a brain tumour and lung cancer about a week after Osh had been born, so the summer of 2021–22 was horrific. I was angry at the world and taking it out on those closest to me. I'd come off the boat and go straight to sleep. When I had my kids with me, the people I treasure most in the world, the noise would be overwhelming, especially over Christmas, the 'happiest' time of the year.

As anybody who has lost a loved one to cancer will tell you, Mum's final weeks and days were ghastly. At night when I was alone in the house with her, all these fears would come. I thought I could ease them with a couple of beers here and there, but hopping off the wagon was a mistake.

When she passed and it came time to plan for her funeral, I couldn't cope. Things were moving too quickly. My sisters were moving through the stages. 'We have to do A, B, C, D and E.'

They would be up to task E and I was still trying to process step A. I couldn't explain how I wasn't coping because I'd just look like a selfish dick. Mum had just died, for Christ's sake. This wasn't about me. I was raised in a place where life revolves around the weather, the grass and the cows. The weather you couldn't do a lot about, and everything else you're bred just to get on with. My sister Becky's in a wheelchair, the result of a car accident in which she was a passenger, and she just gets on with it. So what if I've got a few things going on in my head. I just have to get on with it, too.

Kiko started to get increasingly worried. Again, the specifics of the conversations are gone but she tells me I was talking about not wanting to live.

It was a rough period. There was some chicken-and-egg psychology at play. Was I feeling worse? Was my memory and mood spiralling because I knew I was sick, or because I *was* sick? I still wrestle with that most days.

I still talk to Alix all the time. He reaches out frequently with messages and voice notes. We have plans to do an Ironman together at some point. That will be some achievement: two guys with broken heads encouraging each other around a swim, bike and run course.

I don't know at a personal level if I'm better off with knowing my condition and to some extent knowing my fate, but there is a bigger issue at stake here and it's one I want to continue to be part of. As I've mentioned, my hope is that players of the future don't fall into the same trap I did — that they're not treated like an object and are looked after better by the professional rugby industry.

There needs to be far more support around monitoring head injuries and workloads. It's a conversation that needs to be happening with parents and teenagers at the very start of their prospective careers, not at the end. It doesn't need to be alarmist, but it does need to be honest.

Rugby gave me so much. I saw the world, made lifelong friends, made a lot of money.

It gave me confidence where I might have been lacking it. It taught me leadership and teamwork. It made me physically fit.

Rugby gave me so much, but because I didn't monitor it properly — because I wasn't even aware of the risks involved, which would have enabled me to monitor my brain health more carefully — it has also taken so much away from me.

You can't make rugby totally safe. Accidents are going to happen: legs are going to get broken, knees are going to require reconstruction and players are going to get concussed.

But we need to act urgently to scale down the exposure to the type of subconcussive injuries that are insidious and almost certainly harmful. That means less rugby, for a start. Lower contact areas and less contact training.

You can't see the wood for the trees when you're playing. You talk to any young, aspiring player now and they just want to play, to get amongst it, to prove themselves, their toughness, their skills. If the coach asks them to pack down 20 scrums in a row, they'll do it. If there's a bit of approval at the end of it, they'd do 20 more. That's Pavlovian conditioning.

I played close to 450 games of first-class rugby. It's a number I took great pride in. Now I'd tell you that less is more.

There's a conversation to be had around volume, around exposure to contact. If I can be part of that conversation, then I've achieved something at least in my post-playing career.

4

DUNEDIN, 1993–2000, SOUTHERN MAN

IT'S FUNNY. WHEN I chat to people, many of them assume I spent all my young life in Otago, because they associate me with Otago rugby teams. But if you ask me, I'll say I'm Taranaki through and through. It was never my choice to go to Otago, but Mum and Dad were working towards their dream of farm ownership. A sharemilking opportunity came up in the South Island that brought that dream a step closer to realisation. In an ideal world, they would have stayed on the family farm and worked up to the point of buying it off Grandad. But that wasn't going to happen. Farm inheritance is often a bone of contention, when more than one child enjoys that lifestyle and wants to continue to farm. Mum was obviously pretty keen on the farming life, but so were her brothers. Tradition dictates that the sons usually get first dibs. There's no use in delving into the family politics of it all, but suffice to say it was a bit of a sore point.

The idea was to buy a dairy farm eventually. It was a realistic option back then, but they were already priced out of the Waikato market and Taranaki was becoming more and more unrealistic, too. Land was cheaper in the South Island. Down there, you could get more bang for your buck, so to speak.

So it was off to Otago for the Haymans. It was tough. I was gutted. Coastal Taranaki had been my life and after a rough start, I was really beginning to find my feet at school and in the hostel. I'd got used to the rhythms of boarding school — where to be and when — and was anticipating going nowhere else until I walked out of the gates for the last time. There was a teacher in the PE department called Dale Atkins who was a long-time No. 8 for Canterbury. I'd see him all the time in the gym, and I was looking forward to having his guidance over the next four years. And finally I'd made friends I thought I was going to have for life.

There was a little bit of talk about maybe staying as a boarder at NPBHS and flying south to spend the holidays with Mum and Dad, but I'm not sure it went very far.

There was talk of friends taking turns and driving the tractor down to Otago, but the nuisance value to other motorists would have been extreme, so we utilised the railways for the plant and machinery instead. Mum and Dad hand-picked the best-producing cows from our herd and sold the rest. It's a bit arcane, but if you know your cows, you'll know that the Jerseys are a little lighter-framed so we didn't anticipate they would do as well in the South Island climate. So the best-performing Friesians, or — for the layman — the black and white ones, made the cut. On June 1, 1993, the day that dairy leases traditionally came up, the trucks came, loaded up our remaining herd and headed south to Otago. I travelled in the truck with the cattle. Well, I was up front in the cab, not in the trailer, but you know what I mean. At Wellington, we loaded the cattle onto the *Straitsman*, a livestock ferry, and this was all pretty exciting for a boy just entering his teens whose world until then had pretty much revolved around Taranaki.

I'm fairly sure that was my first trip to the South Island. My first trip overseas. We pulled up at Wyllies Crossing, just out of Mosgiel on the Taieri plains. Wyllies Crossing was just that — an asterisk-shaped intersection where Riccarton Road, on which our property was situated, the Outram-Mosgiel Road and School Road crossed one another. The only other feature of the place was the tiny, one-room school. Like Oaonui, it was the centre of the community and Mum and Dad pretty quickly made friends around the area. Like Oaonui, the school no longer exists as a school, and the building has been converted into a private residence.

There were a lot of lifestyle blocks and smallholdings. We were on one of the few large farms left in the area but we didn't look down our nose at the lifestylers. The opposite, in fact: we came to rely on them due to a series of unforeseen circumstances that had a massive effect on our lives.

There was definitely a settling-in period. We shifted in the middle of winter, and it won't surprise anybody to learn that the biggest difference was the cold. Nobody's going to mistake South Taranaki for Tahiti, but it felt tropical compared to our new digs. Getting into the shed in the morning, if you put your hands on the stainless-steel cups before any milk had gone through, they could stick to your skin like glue — very cold glue. On the farm bike, your hands and feet froze if you were exposed and I'd travel a lot slower to preserve the tyres because the air temperature was so much lower.

I started at King's High School in South Dunedin. I was a day pupil, which meant catching the bus every morning from outside the Mosgiel Returned Services Association. My first full year was fourth form (Year 10, in today's parlance). Any big change at that time of your life is quite daunting. The bus trip was pretty interesting. There was a hierarchy and different cliques depending on whether you were a surfie, a farmer or something in between.

I can't actually remember why I picked King's, although I'm pretty sure it was my decision. We did a tour of the schools. Otago Boys' High had the tradition and the reputation, John McGlashan College had the money and just down the road in Mosgiel, Taieri High School (now known as Taieri College) was far more convenient. Something about King's just appealed to me. It was an all-boys school, although sister college Queen's High was right next door and shared some facilities. It served the more blue-collar areas of the city, like South Dunedin, and it just felt like the right fit.

I arrived in the middle of the footy season — too late to get involved — but I was in time for cricket season. I hauled my gear down there. I still took it really seriously but unfortunately the skills that I thought I had didn't transfer down south as easily as I anticipated. It's fair to say that few at King's will remember me for my feats in whites, despite spending time at the Billy Ibadulla School of Excellence. The former Pakistani Test cricketer and legendary coach had an indoor nets centre near the old Carisbrook ground and I used to go along once a week. I loved it, and really enjoyed my cricket. I desperately wanted to do well but I never really cracked it or even got much of an opportunity.

I thought I could do a job at a higher level than 3rd and 2nd XI with my left-arm medium pacers and hard-hitting, lower-middle-order batting, but it didn't happen. My claim to fame, if you want to call it that, was playing the Otago Boys'

High 2nd XI. OBHS were the flash cricket school on the hill in Dunedin, and they had a young guy called Richie McCaw playing for them. I came in for a flurry late in the innings and ended up hitting four sixes in a row off Richie's bowling. I ended up with about 36 not out. It was on the King's No. 1 field, so there were a few people watching. That was my high point as a King's cricketer.

Have I ever reminded Richie about that day? Yeah, I think it's come up from time to time.

My interest in cricket started to wane when I realised the seconds was my ceiling. The long afternoons became less appealing. It was around this time that rugby started to command more of my attention and time, when off-season training actually became a real thing rather than an idea. Cricket quietly faded into the background and then disappeared altogether. It was a shame, in many ways, but the next Jeff Wilson-style, dual rugby-cricket career was nipped in the bud.

My first footy team at King's was the under-15 Panthers which, along with the Lions — we took a feline approach to grading players — were the school's best teams in that grade. It was such a change from New Plymouth. There, I'd been in the leftovers team, but by the time I weighed-in at King's, I tipped the scales at about 110 kilograms. I was noticed.

I was playing lock. My mate, Warren Moffat — a lawyer, these days, who went on to play more than 200 games for the

Southern club — was also in the team, but we weren't exactly stacked with talent. We were coached by John 'Haggs' Haggart, who was a PE teacher and had played at first-five for Otago. My biggest memory of Haggs was an introduction to the dreaded Hennie Muller drill, where you run the width, length and then diagonal of the field. It was my first introduction to anything that could be loosely called a scientific approach to training. If we — that is, the whole team — didn't complete the distance within a specified time, we'd have to go again. Poor old Moff was a prop who tended to drag the chain a bit, so we'd be trying our best to get him in under the time so we could take a break.

King's had access to some high-profile rugby people. Josh Kronfeld came in to do some work with us. I was playing lock and I remember him saying to me: 'Next lineout, I need you to jump.' I was like: 'I have been jumping!' My aerial ability wasn't quite up to standard, but when you're 14 and 110 kilograms, something has to give. I overheard John Haggart taking Josh aside and whispering to him: 'Josh, that's as high as he can jump. Don't be too tough on him.' He might not have been my biggest fan, but it was pretty cool to have him along. He was already an Otago star and was about to make the All Blacks and revolutionise that openside flanker role.

At the end of that first season, we had a South Island under-15 tournament at Christchurch. We were playing the likes of Shirley Boys' High, Christ's College, Otago Boys' and a few other big rugby schools. Two weeks beforehand, I'd broken my collarbone in a tackle. I'd broken the same bone a few years before playing rugby on the lawn of my grandparents' place with my uncle and a guy called Mark Holmes, who lived across the road and was in the Taranaki under-16 team captained by Reuben Thorne. Well, I spent the two weeks leading up to the tournament trying to convince Haggs I could play, including by hanging off some bars around by the bike shed. I don't know if he could tell that all the force was going through my other shoulder, but he let me travel with the team to Christchurch. I didn't get stripped for the early games, but by the end of the tournament I'd been so persistent that Haggs gave in and let me get stripped to feel part of the team. My shoulder was all padded up. Suddenly, there was an injury to our No. 8. The coach looked to the bench, and a teammate told me to not give him a choice and just run out there. So I did. I sprinted onto the field and packed down at No. 8 before anybody could tell me otherwise. I picked the ball up off the back of the scrum and scored the try, so I had my moment of glory even if, when looking back, it wasn't the smartest thing I'd ever done.

After I broke the collarbone that second time, Mum had had enough. She went to the pharmacy and bought me these calcium pills. They were huge. They looked like they'd been designed for horses, they were so big. I choked them down under her watchful eye, and I don't know whether it was the pills or sheer luck, but that collarbone was the only bone I broke in my entire rugby career, apart from having my nose pushed out of shape a couple of times.

After my exploits for the Panthers, I'd been picked in the 1st XV squad as a lock. It was my third year at high school. The 1st XV coach was Eoin 'Willo' Willis, the father of future All Black hooker Tom Willis: Tom was a year ahead of me at King's. In a coaching sense, Eion was out of the Laurie Mains school: a little bit of a hard-arse. He had these Coke-bottle glasses and a scary demeanour. If he told you to do something, you did it immediately. Nevertheless, Eoin became a mentor to me during my school years, and beyond. He was more than a coach. He was more like a manager. When it came to signing my first contracts for Otago, he was the guy who guided me through the process. Even today he's a close friend, and Tom's a good mate, too.

I'd made no secret of the fact that I wanted more footy than I was likely to get as a reserve lock. One day, Willo took me aside and said that if I wanted to play a decent amount of rugby that year, I'd have more chances at prop than I would at lock. We went over to the scrum machine and he was: 'Rightio, Carl. Jump in at loosehead.' That made sense. At that stage, Craig Dowd was All Black loosehead and a dominant figure in world rugby, and he was tall, just like me. Paul Thompson was another tall loosehead from Auckland, so the thinking was that there was a place for people built like me on the loosehead side of the front row. I had a go on the machine, but it didn't feel right and I wasn't making much of an impression. 'Just pop around to the other side and have a go there,' Willo said.

For the uninitiated, the difference between the 'tighthead' and 'loosehead' propping positions has to do with where your head fits in relation to the heads of the opposing front row when the scrum packs down. The loosehead binds with his head to the left of that of the prop in front of him. His right ear is jammed against the ear of the opposing tighthead, whereas his left ear is in fresh air. His head is said to be 'loose'. The tighthead packs down with his head between those of the opposing hooker and loosehead. Both his ears are jammed up against opposing players': his head is 'tight'.

Honestly, I hit the machine once on the tighthead side and it was like an epiphany. Some things in sport defy rational explanation and this was one of them. Why can some people step up to a tee and with no instruction hit a golf ball down the middle of the fairway, while others can spend years trying to master the game and get nowhere? Why, when everything about my build suggested loosehead prop, did I suddenly find comfort at tighthead? I can't tell you that, but everything clicked. It was an incredible, exciting feeling. I knew it felt good but I also knew that this didn't mean it looked any good. But I looked up at Willo, and he just said: 'That's your spot, there.'

Just like that, on an inspiration from a coach, my fate as a tighthead prop was sealed. If you want to trace the beginning of my professional rugby career, that was the moment. Looking at it in a more macabre way, you can probably trace the start of my head issues back to that moment, too. Twenty years after that first head, I was still throwing my head and neck into scrums and scrum machines, each time pushing the soft jelly of my brain into the wall of my skull, doing damage in imperceptible increments.

So there I was, 15 years old and playing in the local colts competition against 20-year-olds. At that age, even a year's difference can be quite a leap in a physical sense, so I was up against it. These were the days when there were still a bunch of collapsed scrums and neck injuries were an ever-present danger, but I was too young and naïve to worry too much about it. I know Mum and Dad had concerns, though. To give you an idea of the demands of playing in the front row against physically mature young men when you're 15, after my first few games for the 1st XV I'd come home and lie in the bath and Mum would knock on the door to check I hadn't drowned, because I'd have to lie there motionless for a long time before the muscles in my neck and back would unlock enough to let me move. My new role saw me using muscles I never knew I had.

My body slowly adapted to the rigours, but I was aware that what I was doing wasn't normal. It was unusual enough for a fifth former to play in the 1st XV, which was usually the domain of the senior students. But for someone my age to play in the front row was unheard of. I had to admit, it felt good. It wasn't long ago that I'd been a shy and intimidated third-form boarder in New Plymouth, ringing home to Mum whenever I could and playing for a team that was made up of the dregs of those available. Now, here I was, at 15, playing for the 1st XV and hanging out with seventh formers and prefects. There was a sense I'd made it, and even though there was a bunch of boys who had no interest in rugby at all, plenty did. Once I left school, I started to understand how little it all meant, but at the time I was 10-foot tall and bulletproof.

In my first year in the 1st XV, I had Tom Willis next to me at hooker and if he was having a rest it was Greg 'Pos' Gillies, who was as hairy as a possum is furry. Scott Morris, a big redhead, was on the loosehead, or Moff Moffat and a guy called Hamish 'Cat' Caldwell who ended up as a loose forward for the Netherlands but who started out as a loosehead prop. Cat's dad had been a stalwart loosehead for Green Island and also played for Otago, so there was pressure on the son to muscle up in the front row. Poor old Cat would have been lucky if he was 80 kilograms dripping wet. Many years later, he was living in the Netherlands when I was playing for Newcastle. He got hold of me and invited me to his farewell party, which was a game of cricket. We had this proper one-dayer on one of the big grounds in the Netherlands. Chris Williams, another Kiwi who was playing halfback for the Dutch at the time, bowled me a bouncer — or maybe it was a big beamer — but it hit me square in the head. I wasn't wearing a helmet, and I'm not sure if I was sedated by alcohol at that point, but apparently I didn't even flinch and the ball only bounced twice before it crossed the boundary behind the wicketkeeper. The Black Seeds were playing in Amsterdam that weekend, so they came along and you can probably imagine what sort of day it was. There were some people pretty bent out of shape by the end of it.

Elsewhere in the pack we had Johnny 'Muttonhead' Willis. We had some decent backs, like Sam Young, who'd play for Taranaki, but Willo was from the Southern school of coaching and we were a very forwards-oriented, 10-man-rugby type of team. Under the tutelage of Willo and André Bell, who was the backs coach, we had some useful teams, but what has stuck with me longer was the approach to fitness. Being aerobically fit was the be-all and end-all. If you weren't fit, you were of no use to Willo.

The school competition was pretty fierce down south. When we went to Invercargill to play Southland Boys', they had Mils Muliaina and Clarke Dermody. Otago Boys' had Byron Kelleher, Filipo Levi and Richie McCaw, who was a year behind me. We played Shirley Boys' from Christchurch, who had Chris Jack. They were our regular opponents.

In 1997, we made the top four and earned the right to be the sole South Island representative at the nationals. The tournament was at Western Springs, the home of Ponsonby Rugby Club. We were at the tournament with Rongotai College, a boys' school from the Wellington suburbs, Palmerston North

Boys' High and Kelston Boys' High from Auckland, where Ted Henry was headmaster. To say there was a contrast between us and the rest would have been a gross understatement. I'm not going to put this delicately because when you're a schoolboy you tend to say it as you see it, so the truth was Moff was our only player of colour, so we were well below the quota. We lost to Kelston and Rongotai. We'd lost before we got on the field. A lot of our guys were just blown away by the size and physicality of the young Polynesian players. I mean, Kelston had guys who were rumoured to be in the Manu Samoa senior squad.

We didn't do too well, but it was a great experience all the same.

Off the field, family life was becoming a bit more difficult. We literally lived through flood, sweat and tears. The dream of farm ownership died and so, unfortunately, did Mum and Dad's marriage a short time later.

The big wet came first. The Taieri River is an interesting beast. It rises in the Lammerlaw Range, only about 40 kilometres from where it spills into the Pacific Ocean at Taieri Mouth. Despite that short distance, the river travels 288 kilometres in getting there, making it the fourth longest river in New Zealand. It travels north first, into the Rock and Pillar Ranges before turning southeast. It runs through two hydroelectric stations and has cut the spectacular Taieri Gorge before it enters the floodplains where the most fertile farmland in Otago is situated. Much of this area is actually below sea level, and is constantly drained by pumps. Our farm was situated in this swampy catchment area.

There was a big stopbank that ran about a third of the way down our property to protect it from the river. In heavy rain, once the Taieri reached a certain level, the stopbank could be overwhelmed. It had done it most spectacularly in 1980. And then in 1996, it looked like it would do it again.

We had some advance warning that we were about to flood. Dad said there'd been heavy rain up in the headwaters of the Taieri, up in the Maniototo Valley, Andrew Hore country, so we'd better go and move the stock into the third of the farm that was going to be protected by the stopbank.

We got all the cattle to safe ground, but it was touch and go. The water on our property had already risen to the point where we couldn't see any of the creeks that crossed the plain. I had my gumboots and Swanndri on. I was all layered up but ended up walking straight into a creek. With all that heavy clothing weighing you down, you end up scrambling for the side of the creek to haul yourself up pretty quickly. Once we'd finished shifting the animals, I clambered to the top of the three-metre-high stopbank, from which I would normally have a view of the river, 10 to 12 kilometres distant across a grassy plain. Instead, the water was surging past right at my feet, an angry brown torrent that receded to the far horizon.

The stopbank held, and it wasn't overtopped, but all of the grass died. It stank, a really pungent smell of rotting vegetation. Mum and Dad were left essentially milking 300 cows off 100 acres. A healthy dairy ratio is about a cow per acre, so we were well short of that. We became reliant on the goodwill of our neighbours. We'd get calls from all these people on lifestyle blocks saying they had a paddock we could use. For months we'd be walking cattle around the area to graze for half an hour here and there on what was basically people's lawns.

For me and the sisters, it was a bit of an adventure. You'd get out on the farm and help where you could, but for Mum and Dad, it was a time of high stress and massive uncertainty. That dream — obsession, really — of farm ownership would have seemed a lot further away right then. They had no idea it was soon going to disappear altogether.

I guess when you live on a floodplain, you've got to expect to have to deal with the inevitable now and again, but what followed next was entirely unexpected and more devastating. We experienced a once-in-a-generation drought.

It caused enormous strain on everyone. The owner had worked the land himself for years until handing it over to us and he obviously hadn't envisaged living through two years like the ones we had experienced so there was stress on the owner–sharemilker relationship, too.

Mum and Dad were both really hard workers. It's always tough juggling family life with the running of a farm, particularly when circumstances beyond your control are conspiring against you. They would occasionally have workers in to help out, but most of the time it was just them and us kids to help. Dad would pay us $1 per row of milking and $1 to hose down the yards. If I did two milkings a day, I could get $28 — pretty much slave labour, but it seemed a lot to me back then. It wasn't like I had much to spend it on in Ōpunake or Mosgiel, so I used to save it up to buy new cricket gear or some rugby boots.

During haymaking, I'd invite some of my schoolmates from the city out to help. We were still doing some square bales for some horses at the end of the property. Within an hour, all the skin had gone from their hands as they experienced the joys of baling twine for the first time in their lives. They'd all come in shorts, so they had hay splinters all over their thighs. I'm not sure they loved the work, but they loved the feed afterwards. When Mum passed away, I got messages from some of those boys reminiscing about the 'awesome feeds' they were served up after haymaking. If people came to help, the bare minimum was that they went away well-fed. I'm glad they remember that rather than the sores they'd be picking at for weeks.

I never begrudged the work. I never felt like I was missing out on the experiences the townies had of spending lazy days at the beach or the shops. I had an interest in machinery and tractors, so the farm was not just a place of work, but a playground as well. Some of my earliest memories were of

Dad setting me up on the tractor, probably not long after I learned to walk, putting it in low gear and telling me to steer straight for a target in the distance while he fed out the square hay bales. Probably wouldn't get past health and safety in this day and age. From the age of eight, during the haymaking season I'd be set up on the tedder, a machine that cuts and 'wuffles' the hay so it dries quickly before being baled, and away I went. I'd then help Dad turn the hay, so from a young age I had a reasonably mature work ethic. I was exposed to stuff that town kids hadn't even heard of. I learned that if anything broke, you have a go at fixing it yourself before you bring anyone in, whether that's a starter motor on a tractor or a burst PVC water pipe. Farm life taught me that to get anywhere in life, you had to work bloody hard. And seeing the cruel reverses that are part and parcel of primary production probably instilled in me an inbuilt cynicism, too, in that I learned that even if you gave everything to the task, it sometimes wasn't enough.

These factors, a natural work ethic and an acceptance that sometimes there were circumstances out of your control that made a lie of all the hard work you've put in, would help me when it came to coping with the ups and downs of rugby.

Once I left school, I went to Otago Polytech to study. I was playing for Southern by then, one of the great traditional clubs of Dunedin, known for its intense rivalry with Varsity. Willo was coaching there and basically if you didn't go from King's to Southern you would have been disowned. If you look at the title winners over the years, Varsity is miles ahead of the rest and Southern are miles ahead of the third most successful club, Kaikorai.

I played all my rugby with Tom Willis in those early days. We trained together in the gym, getting really serious about it during our last year of school. When we came out of school together we both went straight into the front row of the Southern seniors. We were still basically kids but we were scoring pushover tries and getting noticed in the Dunedin club competition. But with Anton Oliver, Andrew Hore and Eugene Morgan ahead of him in the queue, Tom's path was blocked to the Highlanders. He took an opportunity to go to the Chiefs. I was bloody sad about that, but it was a good move for him. Andrew Hore, who was a great mate of mine, had the same problem. He was trapped behind Anton, so he also moved away to get his shot at playing regularly, in his case to Taranaki and the Hurricanes. It wasn't a situation unique to Otago, but it seemed to happen there more than most: locals who had played all the age-group rep stuff were suddenly bumped when the students came to town. I'm sure there was a bit of resentment, but if you look at it as a whole, the university has been a massive boon for rugby in Otago and players like Anton, who was a Marlborough boy, and Josh Kronfeld from Hastings, were as faithful servants to the blue and gold as anybody who had grown up there.

Playing for Southern was like belonging to an institution. Certain things were drummed into you from the moment you walked into the sheds at Bathgate Park. There were certain games you could not lose and certain ways you had to behave. Our rivalry with University was always top of mind. The two teams played annually for the Vic Cavanagh Memorial Trophy. If you were a Southern man and won nothing else apart from that match, it was still considered a successful season. Another game that was eagerly anticipated for different reasons was the away trip to Eastern. Based in Waikouaiti, the bus trip home involved winding our way down the famous Pigroot Road. It was a pub crawl home through places like Middlemarch and by the time we got back to town we were, to put it mildly, shitfaced.

Steve 'Hotty' Hotton, a tighthead prop and an Otago legend who had his own fan club, was coach. He'd been part of an Otago front row along with hooker David 'Crazy' Latta and the late Steve Cumberland at loosehead. Hotty had a mantra that he drummed into me: you had to train hard, drink hard and win hard games of rugby. I took that advice to heart — too much so, perhaps. Hotty used to pack down in scrums at training and he was the first guy that got super-technical with me at scrum time. He'd tell me if my shoulder was too low here or my back was too high there.

It was an inexperienced side when I joined, with a lot of King's High boys going straight from the 1st XV into the senior squad. We had an English import, Edward Norris, who'd come out to New Zealand for a bit of experience and who had ended up playing for 10 years. It was a great club to be a part of. It had deep connections to the South Dunedin community and saw itself as a home for salt-of-the-earth types, like Mike Reggett, who was groundsman at King's and looked after all the kit and equipment at Southern. There was a couple called Donald and Audrey Todd who'd be at the club, in the same seats, every week. Donald had never played, but the club was part of their identity, so after a game I'd take a jug of beer over to sit with them and have a chat, about life, about footy. I really missed that part of club life when I was playing professionally. While I was still in New Zealand, I tried to make a point of getting back to Southern for one game a year. It got harder and harder, but I'd still go to the club and try to have a presence there.

Donald and Audrey have both passed away now, but when Audrey died, I was sent a folder of newspaper cuttings and photos that she had kept over the years of my career. Some of the hours people donated to that club to look after the clubrooms, the kit or the changing sheds was incredible and really rubbed off on me. Southern used to run the Steinlager tent village during daytime Tests at Carisbrook. That basically bankrolled the club for years. In 2001, I played for the All Blacks versus Australia on Saturday, and on Sunday morning, I was on a forklift stacking pallets and helping clean up. A lot of people mentioned it but it didn't feel like I was doing anything out of the ordinary. It was my club and there was work to do: why wouldn't you help out?

I'd told Reggett when I joined that I was going to be the first player to play 300 games for Southern. I ended up playing 25, so I fell a bit short. I owe him some games but it's true that although I left Southern, the club never left me.

5

MEXICO, 2022, THE TOURIST

WHEN I THINK OF Mexico, the usual clichés spring to mind: hard-shell tacos, cheap Coronas on the beach, crystal-clear waters, spring break and Narcos.

In 2022, I found myself in Monterrey, a huge sprawling city in the northeast of the country, a couple of hundred kilometres from the border with Texas. I was miles from the beach, and beer and tacos were the last thing on my mind.

I was a tourist, all right, but a very modern type — the medical tourist.

* * *

Following my London diagnosis, I fell into a bit of a black hole. There was a lot of stuff going on in my life that I was struggling to cope with and my diagnosis was just part of it. What was I meant to do? Just sit around and wait for my condition to get worse?

Kiko and I were getting frustrated by the lack of support available. I might have been reading too much into it, but there seemed to be a level of cynicism. A kind of: 'Look at the poor former rugby player trying to get a handout' attitude. I didn't want money: I just wanted help with navigating the unknown.

More and more, I noticed that things weren't right. When working on the boat, I couldn't cope with more than a few hours before my body and mind completely shut down, even while doing the most mundane tasks. I was struggling to sustain conversations or trains of thought for any length of time. Even the process of recounting my life for this book was exhausting. My recollections and narration were pretty good and focused for about half an hour. But after that, I'd lose the thread, my responses would get slower and I'd start to veer off on tangents that weren't necessarily related to the subject at hand.

I was getting tired of depression being used as a catch-all to describe my issues. It might not be that sensitive to make a dark joke about it, but it's bloody depressing being told you're depressed every time you need help.

Step forward Alix Popham again. The guy who helped set me up with testing in London put me in touch with another

Welsh guy, Mike Batt, who was on the board of NeuroCytonix, a Monterrey-based biomedical technology company that was developing treatments for neurodegenerative diseases, including CTE. Alix had been twice and was impressed by the improvements the treatments had made to his day-to-day living. I was at a point where I didn't feel like I had a lot to lose, so I paid my money and signed up for a course of treatments.

The trip got off to the worst possible start. Travel had started to make me really anxious, which sounds crazy given how many planes, trains and automobiles I had ridden in since starting my professional rugby career. The process at airports and stations was really starting to freak me out and, sure enough, before we even boarded, my name was called over the speakers because I'd left my laptop, wallet and travel documents at security. Nice work, Carl.

I had brain scans shortly after arriving for my month-long course. It was good to have somebody sit down with me and talk me through them. They didn't sugar-coat it. Whereas the scans in London had picked up two lesions, here they pointed to about 15 microbleeds dotted throughout my brain. The damage was far more comprehensive than I had wanted to believe and fairly sobering.

I read on the internet that in technical terms, a cerebral microbleed is 'a small, chronic brain haemorrhage which is likely caused by structural abnormalities of the small vessels of the brain'. They are most often a consequence of chronic hypertension, cerebral amyloid angiopathy, whatever that might happen to be, and diffuse axonal injury. An axonal injury is the shearing, or tearing, of the brain's long connecting nerve fibres (axons), which happens when the brain is injured as it shifts and rotates inside the skull.

In layman's terms, they show up as black spots on your scan and they're not good news.

Recently, a study funded by the Drake Foundation was published that found that 23 per cent of a group of current elite rugby players were playing with axonal injury or diffuse vascular injury in their brains, while half had unexpected reductions in the white-matter volume, with white matter being the brain's processor. Here I was seeing that in real, not abstract, terms and it was confronting, to say the least.

The doctor told me he wouldn't expect to see a scan like this for a 70-year-old, let alone someone not yet in his mid-forties. While the scans in London had picked up abnormalities, the official designation was that they were unremarkable. Here, the doctor took one look at them and described them as 'truly remarkable'. I'm not sure which was better to hear.

I get asked a bit about all the concussions I received in rugby, and the truth is I didn't have many. There was the knockout blow from Wycliff Palu's head in the Bledisloe Cup Test but other than that, I received very few hits to the head that left me with obvious concussion symptoms.

Subconcussive blows are a different matter, though. Alix reckoned he took 100,000 of these over the course of his professional career. Given my career was longer, I probably took closer to 150,000. Many of these were simply the sort of head-rattlers you get from putting down scrum after scrum against a machine.

To understand what a subconcussive impact is, you need to understand what a concussion is. At its most basic, a concussion is a hit to the brain that causes symptoms that range from being knocked out and unresponsive, to seeing stars and feeling a bit 'spacey'. Concussions have symptoms because the brain is shaken violently enough that cells are damaged to the point where they don't work properly. Subconcussive hits are those that are below that concussion threshold: the brain is shaken, but not so violently that the damage to cells causes symptoms.

Most tackles and collisions on a rugby field, especially those that involve the upper body (as most tackles do these days), will cause subconcussions to both the tackler and the player tackled. The impacts affect the brain: you just don't notice it right away. When I was talking to Chris Nowinski of the Concussion Legacy Foundation, he told me to think about CTE as an overuse injury. Just like a fast bowler in cricket might wear down his back and end up with stress fractures in his vertebrae, a contact sportsman or -woman is continually exposing their brain to microtrauma and CTE might be the result of that microtrauma accumulated over years and years of seemingly insignificant hits. The big difference between a fast bowler and a prop is that he or she can have an operation on their back to fix it. I can't have an operation on my brain to repair the damage.

Because I was worried I wouldn't remember much about the Monterrey trip, I tried to get in the habit of making voice memos. In the past, I might have put it down in emails or even a written diary, but I was beginning to find even that process tiring. I'm basically going to transcribe the memos here, with only light editing to give them a semblance of correct grammar and syntax. By doing this, I hope to paint a real-time picture of what it was like to try both to figure out what was going on in my brain and also find ways of remedying it.

July 4

Travelled down from Los Angeles on a flight leaving around midnight and arriving in the very early morning. I had a few hours to wait for Kiko. It ended up that I was waiting at the wrong terminal, so I had to make my way over to the right one, only to cross paths with Kiko who was already waiting in the car. We got there in the end.

It's nice to be in Monterrey finally. I've been waiting for this for a long time. Monterrey is a city in a hollow so the heat here is pretty extreme.

We settled into a hotel yesterday and had a nice relaxing day catching up on a bit of sleep by the pool before my first meetings at the hospital.

July 5

We were picked up pretty early this morning and went off to the The Center for Research and Development in Health Sciences (CIDICS) at the Universidad Autónoma de Nuevo León, where NeuroCytonix is based. It's centrally based in Monterrey, so was quite a short trip and it's a very modern facility by all standards.

The staff were lovely and very welcoming, spending a lot of time with us today.

Little Genevieve went into the scanner herself as we're a little bit worried she might have a brain condition herself due to her difficult birth, but we'll find out more about that tomorrow.

Then it was my turn. I had an electroencephalogram (EEG) scan to record my brain activity. Sensors were placed on my scalp to pick up the electrical signals produced by the brain. After that I had an MRI. I've spent a lot of time in MRI machines over the years but this one was about an hour and a half. By the end of it I was getting a bit uncomfortable in there and was over it. It was good to get it done.

The staff were really good to us. Even in the conversations I had there today, they were very intrigued to hear about rugby. They don't know a lot about it apart from the haka. A number of the staff asked if I used to do the haka, so it's amazing how that travels and crosses cultures, I guess. It was nice to talk about rugby with them but I certainly noticed that after about 20 minutes talking with them I was starting to struggle to keep up with the conversation.

I had to take a little break, go for a wee walk, take some deep breaths and try to conserve a bit of brain energy for the afternoon.

That's been us really. We checked into our new accommodation; a nice little apartment we've taken near the hospital. We also had our first experience of trying to go shopping. Needless to say we struggled with the language, Spanish is not our strong suit, and with the processes involved. I only lost my gherkin once with Kiko, but she was very understanding. We ended up getting some food, despite it taking a bit longer than normal.

A few feelings that stood out for me. Just realising that I was struggling to follow things in a conversation with three people really stood out. The shopping experience and literally just wanting to get out of the supermarket even before we had everything we needed; I just had this real urgency to get out of there. From here on in I'm sending Kiko to the supermarket and I'll stay here and look after little Bubba Osh.

July 6

Quite a busy day. Out for a little run in the morning to a local park. As I said yesterday, the city is in a big inland hollow so it gets very hot. The traffic is also pretty full on. This city gets to work early and we're right next to a main route so we get a lot of noise here. It was about a 500 m jog to the local park, so it was a lovely way to start the morning.

There was a hospital visit for neuropsych testing and an interview with the neuropsychologist to explain a bit about my background and my history.

We ended at the hospital with my first treatment.

I was pretty anxious today. It was a big, demanding day. The neuropsych test is pretty demanding. Even going into the machine, my blood pressure was taken and it was reasonably high, which is unusual for me because I'm fit and healthy. I guess it shows the anxiety that was building from the morning. It's hard to explain but I just felt off — really anxious, really edgy.

July 7

I feel much better today. Off to the hospital again for some more meetings with doctors and another treatment.

July 9

Just sitting here in a hospital waiting room. I can hear the baby music of Genevieve, who's in the machine in the room next to where I'm going.

I spent a nice morning this morning with Alix Popham and his wife Mel, watching the Wales v South Africa game and couldn't help but think of my current position and the last three to four years, and watching the players on the field and wondering what lay ahead for some of these guys. I've been in that position, where some of those guys are. I gave everything I had to a rugby career and it made me feel a little bit sad. Obviously it won't happen to all of them. It might not happen to any of them, but the chances are some of them are going to have to have issues.

I think about the guys in the era before me too. The guys in their 60s who are having considerable amounts of problems with dementia-related illnesses.

When I thought about it, today was one of the few games of rugby I have sat down and watched in the last three or four years.

Some pretty exciting news this morning. I've been feeling a little bit better and even Kiko mentioned I was contributing a little bit more when we went grocery shopping at the mall. I usually want to get out of there as quickly as possible, but I do feel a small amount of positive change starting to happen, which is awesome news, so I guess we'll see how the next few days progress.

July 10

I'm battling a bit today. We had a dinner out last night with Roberto [Trujillo], who is effectively the lead scientist, the brains behind NeuroCytonix and Alix and his wife and Mike Batt and his wife, plus two of the neurologists here.

The extra activity of trying to follow the conversation has put me in a bit of a weird place today. Everything feels hazy. I feel mentally lethargic. I feel a bit drunk. Everything feels very slow.

Never mind. I'm about to hop in the machine. It'll be coming up a week here soon. I had a little bit of relief yesterday from my headaches and I've had spells of feeling productive again. I even did a few little admin jobs on the computer.

These are little glimpses of me feeling like I can get on top of a few things, so that's really positive.

The after effects of going out last night that I'm feeling today is a timely reminder that I have to look after my brain energy, because it's a bit limited still.

A little bit about this hospital. You make your way down these stairs into an underground level. You'd never suspect that there's potentially life-changing work going on here, behind these little doors. By all accounts there is something special going on here that will help a lot of people. I'm pretty optimistic it's going to help me although a week in, it's been slow progress to date.

July 15

Had a real breakthrough day on Wednesday, with a really clear head. It's the first time in a long time that I've woken up and thought: 'Ooh. I feel normal.'

I had a really, really good day. I'd been expecting it to all come tumbling down at some point but miraculously it didn't.

Sadly, I haven't been able to maintain that over the past couple of days. I had a foggy day on Thursday and here we are on the Friday just before treatment.

I've got some exercise in this morning. We have a lovely park nearby appropriately called Parque El Capitan, so I've been jogging a few kilometres each morning to keep healthy.

The drive to the clinic is quite an interesting journey. We drive through the city alongside big pickup trucks, tiny cars and all sorts of mobiles. Monterrey is quite an Americanised city, which you see in all the pickups and the double-lane motorways that twist everywhere. It's not easy to just get off and on the motorway where you'd like. As we arrive there's this lovely old man who comes out and moves the road cones to let us in and then proceeds to take us through this side entrance, which has wheelchair access because we have Osh in the pushchair.

We could quite easily walk up the stairs and to the main entrance but it'd make us sad not to use his services because he seems to take real pride in helping the funny English-speaking family (and I also think he quite enjoys the chance to get out of the 40-degree heat here, even if it's just for a couple of minutes). Just one of the little slices of life here.

Just heading in for another treatment today and I've just had a phone call from the Concussion Legacy Foundation co-founder Chris Nowinski. He's a former college football player and professional wrestler and it was interesting to have a chat regarding support and things we could potentially put in place for players in New Zealand who will have similar injuries and issues to myself.

As we only have a treatment per day, not to overload myself, but it's been nice to reach out to people, to connect and have a chat around what's on the horizon for TBIs [traumatic brain injuries] and treatment and support. Hopefully there will be some good stuff in the pipeline that we can use for the future.

July 22

Since I last checked in there have been a series of groundhog days, with very similar symptoms and feelings.

I don't have a whole lot to report, really. I have treatment each day and go back to the apartment. I do a little bit of exercise each day to keep things ticking along.

There's been some interesting developments in the head injury department in the past few days with all the news of the red cards and yellow cards. There's also the sad news coming out of England of all the players diagnosed with MND [motor neurone disease], which is obviously pretty sad and heartbreaking for all those involved.

[Note: The player with MND that I am talking about here is Ed Slater, the Gloucester lock who was diagnosed at 33 while he was still contracted to the club. The news story at the time read: 'Gloucester Rugby is deeply pained to announce that Ed Slater has been diagnosed with Motor Neurone Disease (MND). Following six months of testing, Ed's diagnosis was confirmed last week and as a result, with the support of his family, friends and Gloucester Rugby, he has made the difficult decision to retire from professional rugby with immediate effect.' Every story like Ed's feels like a punch in the gut for the sport I love.]

I've been thinking a lot recently about where this is heading with rugby.

I feel looking from the outside that it's certainly giving momentum, the awareness of what's going on with this generation of players and the issues they are facing. Let's hope we can get some support in place for all of these guys sooner rather than later.

Just under two weeks to go now until we head to the UK to see Kiko's family. I am feeling more productive on a daily basis. One of the issues with my situation is that apparently the damage to my brain in one particular part is quite deep, close to the ventricles [large, fluid-filled open structures that lie deep in the brain]. That could potentially take a little bit longer to treat because [the cells in that part of the brain are harder to stimulate]. It might take me a bit longer to feel better like other people who have come through and had the treatment.

Fingers crossed. We're keeping healthy every day and hoping for the best.

July 31

I haven't put together a recording for a number of days. It's been a bit of an interesting week. There's been a stream of articles this week about the legal case I'm involved with against World Rugby. I've been asked to do a few interviews on that at the same time.

That took a bit out of me during the week and I've been struggling since, to be honest. I'm noticing an increased sensitivity to noise. My irritability has increased and has made things a bit interesting for a few days now.

I've been a bit over eager and in terms of results, I've probably expected a bit too much. I had someone explain to me the other day that this is like competing in an Ironman, which I've done a couple of. It's not going to be rip, shit and bust and things happening really quickly. This is going to be a slow process over time.

I do notice that I'm better at times like this, when I'm composing thoughts. I find now that I'm not losing my train of thought as regularly as I used to. Quite regularly I'd be talking and completely lose the thread of what I was talking about or had started saying.

I'm noticing little positive changes and some of that is planning, prioritising relaxation and not taking on too many things at once.

It's been interesting talking to Alix. More than 20 new players in the past few days have contacted him after the news of the class-action case. It's a little bit scary, the magnitude of what's going on here, but I'm really hopeful that new science will really give people a pathway and hope of repairing the damage.

Very interesting times.

I'm looking forward to the end. I'm looking forward to the test at the end of the week and remembering a few more things than normal. I really want those test results to back up how I've been feeling over the past couple of days.

* * *

It's interesting and a little bit sad to read over those transcripts. To see the fluctuations in my optimism and, I guess, at times, my blind faith that I would be 'fixed'.

With the benefit of hindsight, the trip was a rollercoaster.

It certainly wasn't a classic Mexican holiday but there were moments of genuine hope. I recall at one point, Kiko telling me I looked 'radiant', which hasn't been a word used to describe me often.

The 'treatment' that I refer to many times above without describing was an interesting process. I was going to say it was mind-numbing, but the aim was the opposite of that. Essentially, I would show up to the clinic each day and have my blood pressure and vital signs measured. I would be asked a set series of questions, mostly around my headaches and my quality of sleep from the night before.

Then I would lie in this machine. My scans had been stretched onto a transparent sheet that covered my face and helped position me. Then, as it was explained to me, the technician sent a radio frequency into my brain. That sounds a little sci-fi, and perhaps if I had Kiko's natural curiosity, I might have insisted on learning a bit more about the process. I do know it was non-invasive and it wasn't radiation treatment.

I also learned that when you're lying in a machine for an hour a day, alternative rock is not the best choice of music. I quickly changed to something a bit more relaxing and soothing.

So did it work? I think so. I definitely noticed some positive changes that I carried with me long after the treatment stopped.

As I mention in the voice memos, there was one day in particular when I remember waking up and it was a real 'wow' moment. Where was my headache? It was something I'd learned to live with for so long that it was wonderful, yet a little disorienting, to wake up with a clear head.

It was also easier to get a full night's rest. Over time, my sleep patterns had become increasingly disturbed, which had a negative knock-on effect on all the other areas of my life. If I look back to Toulon, when midweek drinking first became a real factor in my life, part of the temptation was that it would ensure I got to sleep, even if I know now that alcohol-induced sleep is of poor quality. Since the Mexico treatment, my sleep patterns have become more normal.

What is slightly harder to measure, and can be a little fickle, is I believe that I have some improvements in short-term memory. When I left the treatment, I was given a document

'CJH Test Cognitivo' that measured my scores from three testing periods from July 6 to the final one on August 2.

The tests administered were:

Montreal Cognitive Assessment Alternative Version 7.2;

Rey–Osterrieth Complex Figure Test;

Trail Making Test;

Symbol-Digit Modalities Test;

Subtests of Wechsler Adult Intelligence Scale;

Rey Auditory Verbal Learning Test;

Boston Naming Test; Stroop Color and Word Test;

Beck Depression Inventory.

When I arrived, my test results showed mild cognitive impairment in the Montreal test and, importantly, 'no clinical depression'.

At the end of my treatment, all my test scores had improved.

Maybe some of the positive outcomes were the placebo effect, or maybe it was because I was coming from some fairly hard work on the boat and the farm I have an ownership share of near Ōpunake. Just being able to decompress, to know that I didn't have anything pressing to do other than check in for my treatment every day, was enough to make me feel a bit more positive about life.

I was living a healthy lifestyle. There was the jogging mentioned in my voice notes, but I also took my bike and would go riding in the beautiful Parque La Huasteca. I even managed to get myself on the back of some group rides and impressed nobody with some pretty average top speeds. I enjoyed Monterrey. It's definitely not what my vision of Mexico was before I left, but we did have some 'authentic' experiences. One of the doctors at the clinic took Kiko, Osh and me to a village on the outskirts of Monterrey, where we ended up at a restaurant eating tacos and other Mexican delights.

I wanted this to work. Even if my melon is too badly dinged up to have a lasting effect, I want places like these to work tirelessly, to research and to test. I'm not naïve. I know for-profit places like NeuroCytonix have a vested interest in being able to show demonstrable improvements in people like me. That's why it's important to have somebody like Kiko by your side. She is more cynical about the medical science industry. She has studied molecular biology at university and her father comes from a medical background. She questions everything. When it comes to medicine and 'miracle treatments' her rule of thumb is: 'Things that sound too good to be true usually are.' I probably operate more on feelings. It felt good to wake up without a headache, even if it was just for a day. It felt good to be a little sharper in testing, to feel slightly more 'on to it' on a daily basis.

One of the questions Kiko asked was particularly relevant. The treatment I was receiving was all around the stimulation of cells in areas where there was noticeable damage to my brain —

around the bleeds. CTE, on the other hand, was the collection of tau protein in the crevices of your brain matter. The tau molecules, whose function — ironically — is to protect brain cells, had detached from microtubules to form long filaments, or neurofibrillary tangles, that disrupt the brain cells' ability to communicate with other cells.

So the stimulation of my brain cells was great, but what could we do to slow down, disrupt or even break down the neurofibrillary tangles?

As I write this, I am part of a London-based clinical trial for a drug that aims to break down these tau protein tangles and excrete them from the body. We were introduced to the trial by Dr Emer MacSweeney, a neurologist who recently gave a TED Talk entitled 'CTE: The silent killer in contact sports'.

In introducing her subject, MacSweeney said: 'Despite the 2013 landmark multimillion NFL settlement for retired American football players with brain injury and the 2015 Will Smith movie *Concussion*, the fear and reality of dementia in contact sport is still not widely known, it is still not adequately addressed and it is not going away. We rely on experts to identify and explain these risks, but many have downplayed the reality. Consequently, too many players, coaches, parents and fans remain unaware of what is now known.'

Couldn't have put it better myself.

The drug I am on at the moment has been shown to have had a remarkably positive effect on patients with frontal-lobe dementia and it is hoped the effect will be similar for those suffering from probable CTE. I'm certainly hopeful it will have a positive effect on me. It's early days but I don't mind sharing one of the immediate by-products of the drug. It makes your pee turn blue, which in turn makes it impossible to get away with leaving the seat down when you go to the loo.

When I think about the treatment I had in Mexico and the positive offshoots of that, and this trial I am on at the moment, I find I have a twofold motivation. Obviously, first and foremost, I want a cure. If the medical science community can find some way to rid the brain of the harmful protein that collects and disrupts cognition, that would be the ultimate.

But there's something else at play here. A very simple word. Hope.

I want players like me, whether it's rugby, football, American football, the AFL or whatever, to feel that a shattering diagnosis such as the one I received isn't the start of a grim final chapter of their lives.

Because sometimes that's how I feel: hopeless. And it's not a nice place to be. Hope is much more welcoming.

6

ALBANY, 2000, ALL BLACK #1000

ONCE I CONVERTED TO the front row, things started falling into place for me in age-group rugby. I'm not sure if you could say I was on a fast track to the All Blacks but things started moving pretty quickly — probably too quickly — once I started playing senior rugby. Previously, I made the New Zealand Under-16s and spent two years in the New Zealand Schoolboys side. Some of the other guys in the 1996 side who went on to play for the All Blacks were the hookers Andrew Hore, who captained the team, and Keven Mealamu, while Doug Howlett and Kevin Senio were in the backs. The following year, we had a bigger programme of matches and the team included Clarke Dermody, Ross Filipo, Campbell Johnstone and my King's mate Tom Willis, all under a hard-nut captain out of Wellington called Jerry Collins. Joe Schmidt was one of the coaches of the team.

If you graphed my rugby trajectory alongside my academics, you'd have seen them heading in opposite directions. The scholarly side of my life had tailed away. I'd done all right at School Certificate in fifth form (or Year 11), but things went downhill the following year, and in my final year of school I was doing a sports performance course rather than anything curriculum-based. I wasn't dumb, but I didn't put the time into my subjects that I needed to. You offer me the option of a gym session or hovering over my books, and I was choosing the weights every single time. I wish I'd done more at school and the smart thing to say here would be that I regret it and put out a public service message like: 'Kids, listen up in school', but the truth was that I recognised even back then that being rugby smart and farm smart was probably going to be more applicable to my life than being book smart.

Tom Willis was doing the sports course, too. He was a really smart student, and had already done seventh form (Year 13), but returned to school so he could go on the tour with the New Zealand Secondary Schools. It meant we got to spend a few hours each day training. We were effectively living a professional sports life before we knew what one was.

That's when I realised that as much as I loved playing rugby, I really, really loved training. That work ethic and desire to push myself in the gym never left me during my career. It gave me an edge over players who loved the game, but couldn't really be arsed with everything that came with it.

Along with representing New Zealand at schoolboy level, I also made the Under-19s and Colts. I made the latter team as an 18-year-old, so had three years with them, which was fairly rare. It meant I was on the national selectors' radar, but my age-group status didn't cut much ice when it came to senior rugby. It was still daunting as an 18-year-old front-rower turning up to training and going shoulder-to-shoulder with tough men who had loads more experience than I had.

At that time, it was still a huge deal to play for your province. Super Rugby hadn't become the all-dominant competition below Test rugby. Making the Otago side was fiercely competitive and a source of huge pride. Look at the front row alone, with guys like Anton Oliver, Kees Meeuws, Carl Hoeft and Joe McDonnell. Great hookers like Tom and Andrew Hore were Otago men through and through, and had to head off elsewhere to get NPC game time. To be invited to training and rocking up into that environment as a teenager was frightening. I knew guys like Taine Randell and Josh Kronfeld were intense, demanding characters when it came to training, so it's no exaggeration to say I was more worried about footy practice than I was about games in those early days. Plus

I'd already had a punch-up with Joe while playing a club game for Southern against his Zingari-Richmond team. He gave me a cauliflower ear on the first scrum and kept boring in so we came to blows. It was a bit of harmless handbags but I knew at an Otago training there'd be that type of intensity from everybody and I spent the day before my first practice shitting myself about what was to come.

There were a lot of the All Blacks in the team who would miss big chunks of the season, so the idea was for me to be primed to potentially fill in for Kees, either as a starter or off the bench, when he was away.

My starting debut in the National Provincial Competition came against Waikato at Carisbrook. Across the line from me was loosehead prop Michael 'Meat' Collins, now CEO of the Chiefs. I had a reasonably good game scrummaging-wise, but you only have to get one wrong for it to be the only thing people will remember. Inevitably, there was one scrum where I got my angles slightly wrong and Meat shot me out the roof, so to speak. That's a no-go as a tighthead: you're standing straight up as the rest of the scrum remains packed around you, a fairly ignominious way to mark my big day.

You have to cast your mind back to remember what the National Provincial Championship (NPC) was like. I remember playing Canterbury on the 'Brook in an NPC game and there were 25,000 people there, mostly screamingly drunk students. In the late '90s, a lot of guys in the team were still students and most of us were flatting. It's probably an exaggeration, but it felt like somebody in every flat in Dunedin had a connection to someone in the Otago team. The support from the student body was both organic and meaningful. It didn't matter where you came from in the country, when you came to Dunners, you bought a blue and gold jersey or a scarf.

Slowly that changed. When professionalism took hold properly, we lost our connection to the student population. Students from out of town brought their allegiances to the teams representing the places they were from. Even as I made my debut, the Super 12 was on the rise, and was beginning to take over. It wasn't necessarily a good thing. By the time I left in 2007, we'd be lucky to get three or four thousand along to our NPC games.

Sadly, now, I don't think many come into town supporting any NPC team and even the support for Super Rugby seems pretty tepid in comparison.

My memory of those early forays into provincial rugby are either blurry or gone altogether. I'd struggle to tell you about tries scored or matches won and lost, but I can remember little incidents that added to my understanding of what it meant to play senior provincial rugby. One lesson involved John 'JL' Leslie, an experienced campaigner in the Otago midfield. It might have been the game against Waikato — doesn't really matter, but what he said did. During a stoppage in play, he came running over and gave me a serve in front of everyone because one of their players had been caught on the wrong side of a ruck and I'd stepped over him, not on him. He let me know in no uncertain terms that if they were stupid or cynical enough to be on our side of the ruck, I was obliged to jump all over them. You couldn't do that now. It's an almost unrecognisable game in that respect, but deliberately rucking an opponent wasn't just accepted back then: it was expected.

Shit, there was some experience in that 1998 team. That first-choice front row was incredible. The loosies were dominant. Simon Maling was a good mate and a lock who was both athletic and a great lineout technician. We had glue guys — players who did their jobs in an unfussy way and allowed others to shine — like Brendon Timmins, John Blaikie and Kelvin Middleton, who might not have played for the All Blacks, but knew their way around a rugby field. Kelvin was married to Rachel Hunter, the daughter of legendary Otago coach Gordon Hunter. Gordie lived two doors down the road from Mum and Dad — the back-to-back effects of the flood and drought had meant they could not make a go of the farm, so they gave up their lease and moved into Dunedin — so we got to know the Hunters well.

The backs were a flasher type of human than the forwards, but there was a nice mix of locals and blow-ins, with Byron Kelleher at halfback, Tony Brown at flyhalf and the talents of Romi Ropati, John Leslie, Brendan Laney and Jeff Wilson around them.

We won the NPC that year, thrashing Taranaki in the semi-final and Waikato in the final. We were ridiculously dominant.

Anton summed it up when he said: 'I can't recall, before or since, having played with a pack that was regularly as efficient, skilled and ruthless all round. And our backs were also skilled and penetrative all year... crucially our reserves were talented, resolute and reliable.'

'Resolute and reliable.' I'd have taken that at that stage in my career — or at any stage, for that matter.

There was some irony in that the year of dominance for Otago with an All Blacks-laden team, came against the backdrop of one of the worst, if not *the* worst, years for the national team under the coaching of John Hart and captaincy of Taine Randell. They lost five Tests in a row and Taine's leadership — he was a relatively young captain in a team with some dominant, hard-headed personalities — came under intense scrutiny.

Taine was a big thinker when it came to rugby, a fine athlete around the field and a formidable lineout forward at No. 8. I felt for him, because he copped a lot of grief. His captaincy also coincided with an era when Australia was chock-full of great, intelligent players like John Eales, George Gregan and Stephen Larkham. I'd watch Taine play for the All Blacks and it didn't look like he was enjoying himself. Still, he never brought that angst back with him to Otago, and even if he had, we were like a family and would have wrapped our arms around him. I can't emphasise that enough. That Otago team was way more than a sports team. One of the worst days of my rugby career was my final game for Otago after I'd signed overseas. I came off the field and just broke down and cried. It was one of those, 'Shit. What have I done?' moments. I was a rugby mercenary from that moment forward. It didn't mean I wasn't going to give it my all, but I was playing for money, not for the people and the place. Otago had been such a massive part of my life. And sure enough, I had a great time elsewhere, but I never again replicated that passion I had for Otago. I grew to really like Newcastle and I probably ended up loving Toulon, but there was still not that raw passion. The love I had for Otago and the Highlanders ran deeper. It never felt like a job, not once: it was a way of life.

Tony Gilbert, who was coach in 1998 before taking the Highlanders job the following year and joined Wayne Smith's All Blacks coaching panel a year later, was instrumental in forging that passion. He was like the godfather of Otago rugby — a benevolent one, not the kind from a Francis Ford Coppola movie. He was an amazing people-person. I firmly believe if he had stayed with the Highlanders and not gone off to the All Blacks, he would have created a dramatically different rugby landscape down south and we would have avoided the dramas that were to follow. His shoes were too difficult to fill. He was a great facilitator. In Tony Brown and Taine Randell, he knew he had super-sharp rugby brains on the field for him, so he played more of an overseer's role.

He was pivotal to that 1998 NPC success, but he couldn't transfer that success with Otago to the All Blacks. I don't want to belittle him or say he wasn't up to international coaching standard, because he definitely was, but the feedback I got was that some of the players, particularly from Auckland, didn't really rate him. My guess is they were used to coaches who told them what to do, but Tony wasn't really like that: he preferred his players to figure it out and gave them the tools to think for themselves. It's pretty common practice these days, but back then that kind of player empowerment was pretty radical, and if you weren't used to it, there was a chance you could come across as a coach who was indecisive or not prepared to take responsibility.

We rated him, though. We loved him.

They were exciting times for me off the field, too. I had gone flatting in Park Street in North Dunedin, very close to the 24-hour dairy where all the students hung around after a big night drinking. I was loving the independence, but it was also handy knowing I had Mum and Dad not too far away if I needed a bit of home cooking. I was flatting with Moff and a few girls and was studying at the Sports Institute. The institute was part of the polytech, but based out at Mosgiel, so I'd drive out there every day. The former Otago player John Haggart was at the institute and was looking after the rugby players, along with a guy called Murray Roulston, who was one of the first coaches to break down the constituent parts of rugby into very specific skill requirements. I didn't realise how influential this was to me at the time.

Until Roulston started getting into the minutiae of the game, rugby coaching had been quite generic. But here was a guy getting super-specific about every skill, every angle, every muscle I'd need. Some of the stuff he said still sticks with me today. He'd tell me that he didn't care if I was a tighthead prop: I still needed to learn how to follow through with my leg to give the ball more chance of sitting up when performing a grubber kick. I became known, I guess, as a skilful operator in the front row — not through kicking, it should be noted — and it was Roulston who planted the seed that skills were as important as brute strength and physicality.

Another guy, fitness trainer Matt Blair, was important in my journey to understand that lifting heavy wasn't the be-all and end-all at that age. Lifting weights correctly and having good technique was more important than just getting in the gym and smashing out huge numbers and lifting as much tin as I could. The temptation was to go in, throw as much as you could on the squat bar and grunt, but Matt, who we used to call 'Form' because everything was about keeping your form, would tell you to put 80 kilograms on and get used to lifting that comparatively light weight properly. Jeremy Stanley got to know Form at his finest and most pedantic when he came down from Auckland and went to his first fitness test. The test included 30 chin-ups, which Jeremy quickly popped out, only for Form to tell him to grab the bar and start again. He refused to count them until Jeremy started straightening his arms. Form was Form: a lovely man, but very strict, as Jeremy found out to his cost. For an 18-year-old full of testosterone, Form saved me a lot of injuries over the course of my career.

I often think about how fortunate I was to run into the right people at the right time of my career. There was Willo, who was the perfect schoolboy mentor, teaching me that nothing you want badly enough comes easily in life; Murray Roulston, drilling down into technical detail when I was a sponge who wanted to learn; Form, who taught me how to lift properly before bad habits of the kind that I've seen sidetrack careers slipped in; and later Mike 'Cronno' Cron, who perfected the angles and body positions required to make scrummaging an art form.

I was a young kid who was pretty strong and robust. I had the raw mechanics, but you need so much more than that to refine yourself into a professional player.

At Otago, we didn't do a lot of live scrummaging at training. We had this old wooden scrum machine. I can still picture it now. You hit it the first few times in pre-season training and it sent a rattle through your entire body. In my mind's eye, I can still see the evil thing sitting there in the paddock. There's no 'give' in it: just a couple of flimsy pads on a wooden sled. No springs, just pure resistance.

I'm going off on a tangent here, but that Otago scrum machine wasn't the worst I'd encountered. There was a session I did once for the Southern Region schools team under the eyes of Gary 'Chainsaw' Lennon, an old master from St Bede's in Christchurch. Chainsaw was an interesting character. He had this team speech where he'd go around the team and in this inimitable voice, tell you what you had to do in the game. 'Hayman. Push hard in the scrums and get around the field,' he'd say. 'Tom Willis. Get your throws to the lineouts on target, hook the ball cleanly and make your tackles.' He did this for every player in the team until he got to the fullback.

'Ben Blair,' he said, before pausing. 'My wife likes little boys like you, Ben.'

I remember it clear as day now. At that stage, Ben was seen as the next Jeff Wilson. He was really good at cricket as well as rugby and had this amazing, left-foot step. Ben waited on further instructions, but that was all Chainsaw had to tell him. The look on Ben's face was priceless — mostly confusion with just a hint of fear.

Chainsaw took us to St Bede's in Christchurch for a training session. They had this scrum machine under the gymnasium on a wooden slat floor. We were doing this scrum session in this small, enclosed area with a machine that had no give on a slat floor that meant you had to place your feet precisely or you'd trip yourself and everyone else up. The scrum machine itself was a piece of shit, all steel and wood with this pointless leather covering. It was like scrummaging against concrete. It was one of the worst training experiences of my life and I came away with these huge, bloody welts where my skin had stretched and bled underneath. It was dreadful, but at 16, you're just a big kid and Chainsaw was quite a scary figure, so of course, you didn't say anything. It was pretty barbaric. I'm not sure if St Bede's has produced many All Black front-rowers, but if they haven't, I think I know why.

When I look back at my career, I realise just how much of my early days at Otago I spent just existing. Unless you were an extremely confident young player, like a Jeff Wilson or a Josh Kronfeld, the thought of adding something to the team environment other than your ability to follow orders and instructions just wouldn't cross your mind. I was in that Otago team purely to make up numbers. I was a body. A big body. That was the sum total of my input.

I had size and a reasonable amount of fitness, but I was running on excitement and fear rather than any guile or knowledge. I was using far more adrenaline than I was brain cells. My mental state changed as I got older. When I was younger, it was all about effort. As you get older you think more technically; you play with the same intensity, but with what sports psychologist Gilbert Enoka calls a 'blue head' — with the calm, rational part in control. When I was younger, I played with a 'red head': I had tunnel vision and went at things like a bull at a gate. I don't mean this to sound arrogant, but later, at Toulon, I would sometimes surprise myself at just how clearly I saw the game. I'd literally be deciding what I was going to do in a few phases' time. The game was beautiful. It was in slow motion. I was making calculated decisions and I'd chuckle at some of the young players huffing and puffing here and there and achieving far less in the process. 'Jesus,' I'd think to myself, 'is that what I used to look like in my Otago days?' No doubt it was.

As a player, I had two strings to my bow. I set a steady scrum and I became known as one of the better 'lifting' props. This wasn't really a skill I learned at school because my height meant I was used extensively as a lineout forward, jumping almost unopposed at number one in the lineout. It was a sound tactic. Most of the props standing next to me were five-foot-four so if you just threw the ball to me at the front of the lineout, it was pretty easy to win the ball without too much resistance.

Once I started lifting, that height and strength gave me obvious advantages. It's a matter of long levers and getting my jumpers up there a bit longer and a bit higher. I put a lot of thought and work into it, to the point where we were experimenting with one-man lifts.

Having made Otago as a teenager and the Highlanders shortly afterwards — 1999 was the year of the 'Party at Tony Brown's' loss in the final to the Crusaders, and the following year we lost convincingly to the same team in the semi-finals — my next big break came when I was picked for a New Zealand A tour to Europe.

The team was coached by Robbie Deans, with Steve Hansen as one of his assistants and Darren Shand the manager. There was some real experience in the playing group, with Tony Brown at first-five joined by the likes of Mark 'Sharkey' Robinson, Rua Tipoki and Scott McLeod in the backs. There were some old stagers like Slade McFarland and Con Barrell alongside me in the front row.

It was a fun tour, though the itinerary was a bit weird. We started in Lens in the industrial north of France for a game against the French Barbarians. That part of the country is not really known for rugby — it's a big football and cycling region — but we thought we'd head out on our first night in town and try to chat up the local girls. Sharkey was probably doing better than most, but someone slipped him a sleeping pill and stole his false tooth. He didn't take it very well and the following day Shand had to make a plea to the rest of the team for the culprit to return his tooth, because Sharkey was about to pack his bags and fly home.

The tour was a lot of fun. I was green as grass, and in that first match we came up against what was effectively a shadow French team. We got towelled up front, coming up against a front row including Pieter de Villiers and Christian Califano. The Barbarians won that game 23–21, but we had more joy the following week in Cardiff, where we beat Wales A 30–9.

From there we headed down to Bayonne, where we beat France Universities comfortably enough. Bayonne is right next door to the Basque seaside city of Biarritz, where I celebrated my twenty-first birthday. Not a bad spot to bring up a milestone.

They were running this tour concurrently with an All Blacks tour of France and Italy, and two days after we beat France Universities, the All Blacks got hammered by Les Bleus in Marseille. It was the second Test of the series — the All Blacks had won the first in Paris — and Greg 'Yoda' Somerville had been injured in the process. I'd received positive reviews for my performances on the A tour, so I was pulled from New Zealand A and flown to Genoa in Italy as cover for that Test. Gordon Slater, another man of good Taranaki farming stock, was first in line to replace Yoda, but if the Cantabrian didn't recover, there was a chance I might get a spot on the bench. As it happened, the injury can't have been serious because I hadn't been in Italy long before I was put on another plane to rejoin the As, this time in… Bucharest.

Romania actually has a pretty proud rugby history, having beaten many of Europe's top teams, including several wins against France. Under Communism, the sport was strong amongst the military; but the end of the Iron Curtain and dictatorial rule hadn't been good for Romanian rugby. In fact, when we travelled there, neither the country nor the team was in great shape.

Everything about Bucharest was so grey and bleak. Every apartment seemed to have washing hanging from the balconies and on the bus on the way to practice, we took to counting the stray dogs. We got to 50 one day before calling it quits. We smashed Romania 82–9 in front of bugger-all people, and it felt a very flat way to end my first international senior tour. I was more than happy to get on the plane and get out of there.

The tour gave me a lot of confidence. While I was loving the environment with Otago and the Highlanders, they were so strong in those days that I felt like I was playing a bit part. In those initial Super 12 campaigns in 1999 and 2000, I was very much the new blood, taken along to get 20 minutes here and there. Making the New Zealand A team and then playing well — well enough to get a call-up to the All Blacks, even if it was more through circumstance than anything else — was a boost to my self-esteem. I knew I hadn't 'made it', but I also knew that the progress I was making was being recognised.

In that respect, 2001 was a breakout year for me. Peter Sloane had replaced Tony Gilbert as Highlanders coach and there was a good atmosphere at the team. I was still a long way from the back of the bus in terms of team hierarchy (it's a long-standing tradition that the senior players get to sit at the back of the bus), but I was starting to get the No. 3 jersey ahead of Meeuws. I wasn't a big follower of the media, but I started to pick up on chatter that I might make the All

Blacks. I did read newspapers, but I never sought one out to read about myself. I felt that if I was going to read the papers when I was going well, I should read them when I was going badly, and I really didn't want to do that in those early seasons of Super 12. I knew I might not have liked what I saw.

I still didn't back myself, and when you're going to play in South Africa in those big rugby cathedrals, against players like Os du Randt, Ollie le Roux and Daan Human, if you doubt yourself, you're in trouble. In 1999, I was called over to South Africa and took the bench against the Sharks at Kings Park. Sure enough, I got on the field and there was a scrum and I found myself looking across at Le Roux, a 130-kilogram concrete block of a man. You can't help but think, 'What the fuck am I doing here?'

Those South African stadiums were so intimidating. The crowd was close, the stands were steep. When you're sitting with the reserves, you're getting dog's abuse from behind you. It was probably better at places like Johannesburg, Pretoria and Bloemfontein, because the crowd would be speaking Afrikaans. You didn't know what they were calling you, but you had a pretty good idea it wasn't: 'Hello, Carl. You seem a nice fellow. Good luck for the game!'

The more I was exposed to those South African teams in particular, the more confidence I started to get. That's when, I guess, the ABs talk started in earnest.

Dad was hearing it, too, maybe through Gordie Hunter, who was pretty crook with cancer by then, but still had his ear to the ground concerning matters of national importance. Dad would take Gordie out on his boat in the harbour. They were fishing for salmon but seemed to catch a lot of sharks, too — more than enough to convince me it wasn't a great place for a swim.

Dad decided not to pass on any of the rumours, which was probably a good thing, saying he didn't want to build up my expectations and then let me down. But talking to him later, it was clear it was more not to build up his own expectations. He never said a lot, but the old man was proud of the way my career was tracking. He had come on a tour to South Africa with the Colts one year and he and Paul Tito's dad certainly took advantage of the country's legendary hospitality.

In 2001, the first All Blacks squad was named to face Manu Samoa, Argentina and France. This was a curious era — mobile phones and the internet were around, but most people still found out about the team by listening to the radio. I was around at Mum and Dad's when the team was named. Just like that, there was my name. It was a surreal feeling, but there were no great celebrations, as I recall. I do remember whatever emotions I felt pretty quickly circling back to fear. How many 21-year-old All Black props were there? Are they really sure I'm good enough for Test rugby?

I got a call from somebody at New Zealand Rugby. I couldn't tell you who it was, but they told me to get myself down to the Leisure Lodge in North Dunedin to do some media. I can't remember what I said. It wouldn't have been much, but I do remember a few sideways glances as I turned up in my brown woollen jumper, old footy shorts and socks and jandals. Being a young fella, I didn't put too much thought into what I should wear for the occasion. Even if I had thought to change, I'm not sure my wardrobe was extensive enough to paint me in a more flattering light. I suppose I probably could have mustered up a pair of jeans and some shoes if I'd known they wanted me to look flash.

Don't ask me to recall much about the lead-up to my first Test or even the Test itself. I can tell you the game was at Albany, at North Harbour Stadium, against Manu Samoa, and that we stayed at the Poenamo Hotel in Northcote, which was still the tradition for the All Blacks back then. We walked across the road to training at Onewa Domain, or maybe it was Hato Petera College.

I have no memory of the game apart from running on to replace Yoda with about 20 minutes to go. I know we won comfortably, 50–6, in a pretty ordinary performance, and I know that when I took the field, I officially became the 1000th All Black. Nothing else sticks about that first week.

There was no big induction ceremony that I recall, and this might sound weird, but I have no recollections of Wayne Smith from that time. He was the head coach. When I think about him now, my memories are all from that 2004–07 period, when his analysis seemed so far ahead of anybody else — always on point and easily understood. Yet here he was, my very first All Black head coach, and when I reach back into the memory banks, I can't find a thing to cling to.

Tony Gilbert was the forwards coach and I loved the bloke. I found him really honest and relatable. As I've said, he didn't get the same buy-in from the guys from outside Otago, which was a real shame. When I think about the roles Tony and Wayne had, I reckon they would have had more chance of long-term success had their roles been reversed, because Tony was more an overseer, and Smithy was better at getting into the weeds when it came to tactics and technique. Smithy would have been a great foil for Tony, rather than the other way around.

At that stage, we were having massive lineout issues. Anton Oliver was copping a lot of flak for his throwing, but I found that strange because I knew Anton was a bloody good thrower. At Otago, I lifted guys and it was a rare lineout when Anton failed to throw darts right into their hands at the top of the jump. We never had timing issues at the Highlanders, but it was a different story with the All Blacks.

The biggest reason, I suppose, was the fact that we were regularly playing the two best lineouts in the world in the Springboks and Australia. The Wallabies could throw up John Eales, Justin Harrison and Owen Finegan, and the Boks — with Victor Matfield, Mark Andrews and André Venter — were possibly even better. We had good players, like Troy

Flavell, Taine, Reuben Thorne and particularly Chris Jack, but our lineout was miles behind the other Tri Nations outfits. Lineouts are truly a team effort, and ours was lagging.

The scrum was much better, with Carl Hoeft, Anton and Yoda the preferred starting front row. Hoefty liked to tick off the tightheads he came up against and, by his judgement, got the better of. The only name I recall that he never felt he got the better of was Springbok prop Cobus Visagie, who got busted for steroids but later on, so Hoefty gave himself a free pass for that.

I have to be honest and say the All Blacks environment was a disappointment and a bit underwhelming. I was young and ready to soak it up, but the culture we had at the Highlanders felt more conducive to good footy than the All Blacks. It felt like people were looking after their own interests more than those of the team — not on the field during the games, so much, but around the camp.

We had Mike Cron as scrum coach. He was an absolute genius, but some of the older guys didn't want to listen to him. They didn't buy into his methods. It was a bit like with Tony Gilbert: they were used to doing things a certain way and were resistant to change.

There was quite fierce internal competition for some spots. These were the days when rugby was still largely considered to be a 15-man game rather than the 23-man game it is now, so winning a starting spot was all important. Nowhere was that tension more obvious than at halfback, where Justin Marshall and Byron 'Wazza' Kelleher, two fiercely competitive individuals, were fighting for the No. 9 jersey.

Marshall had the game nous and experience but Byron probably offered a bit more physically at that point in their careers. I'd come through the grades watching Wazza. He was older than me, so I never played him at school, but I remember watching him play for Otago Boys' against King's one day. At that time, we had a No. 8, Paul Miller, who was a high-school juggernaut. He used to score these amazing, long-range tries and probably thought he was set for another one when he cleared out against Otago Boys'. Next thing you heard was this almighty thud as Wazza did what none of the forwards had successfully managed and picked Paul up and dropped him on his arse with a crash.

Wazza was a real character. He got his nickname because at his first Otago training, Josh Kronfeld asked him what his name was and he had his mouthguard in and Byron came out sounding like Warren. He wasn't always the sharpest tool in the shed, and took so much stick from teammates, but sometimes I think it was an act and that he liked people underestimating him.

He was also a guy who had no shame. Darren Shand loved him because when Wazza was on the entertainment committee, he'd have no problems going to restaurants he liked the look of and asking for a free team meal in exchange for gifts of jerseys and photos they could hang on the wall. It'd save Shandy about $40,000 in expenses per year. He was the opposite of me like that. I could never ask anything of anyone and, as a result, never took advantage of any sponsorship opportunities.

When we were staying in Aix-en-Provence at the 2007 World Cup, we had a day off and Wazza and Dan Carter went to nearby Monaco, where they met Prince Albert. Wazza later ended up being a guest at the Prince's wedding — although, knowing Wazza, he probably invited himself.

Wazza became a bit of a god in Toulouse, where he played from 2007 to 2011. After he retired, he set up a bar there, the Haka Corner, which was designed to be like the All Blacks' changing shed. I went to the opening of the bar and had a great night, but I don't think New Zealand Rugby or Māori leaders were too impressed with the concept.

Life was never dull with Wazza around, but a bit like me, he has made the news for all the wrong reasons in recent years, with alcohol at the root of most of his notoriety.

My first start in an All Blacks jersey came a week after my debut, when we met Argentina — Los Pumas — in Christchurch. They were known as one of the better scrummaging nations, and there was even a specific term for their technique in this area: the 'bajada' or 'bajadita'. The method was developed in the 1960s by Francisco Ocampo, and it basically means an eight-man shove where all their collective power is directed through the hooker. The other defining characteristic is the 'Empuje Coordinado' or co-ordinated push, where they breathe in, breathe out and push in unison.

Some of their advantages in the scrum had been nullified to an extent by the 'crouch, touch, pause, engage' rules that were brought in, but in Roberto Grau, Omar Hasan and Federico Mendez, they had a formidable front row. On the bench, they could call on Mario Ledesma and Mauricio Reggiardo, so it was shaping up to be a long night. We were staying at the Heritage Hotel in Christchurch, right on the Square, and I spent a bit of time that week staring out the window, wondering what I had got myself into.

It was such a long week. Mike 'Cronno' Cron, the scrum coach, was stoking the fires and I caught a bit of the news that claimed the Argentine front row were wanting 'to scrutinise Hayman's technique'. It was the most apprehensive I've ever been. On the evening of the game, I was getting so anxious that I felt like I was short of breath. I had to lie on the hotel room floor to get some deep breaths in before I went down to get on the team bus.

Night rugby is such a part and parcel of the modern game in the southern hemisphere that it is probably hard to comprehend now, but in those days we had to put a lot of thought into how we were going to manage game day. We were looking for the perfect formula that would allow you to switch off and not overeat, which was always a battle for someone like me, who's quite fond of their food. Do you drink coffee, go for a walk, watch movies? I tried a lot of different stuff, but what I kept coming back to, what helped me relax the most, was a good stretching session. If you feel limber and loose, it loosened up your mind, and the opposite was true if you were tight.

Conrad Smith, myself, the physio Pete Gallagher and Keven Mealamu decided to start baking it into our game-day prep and pretty quickly we had even the cynics joining us in our 'Stretchercise' classes. It became an organic hit within the squad. I could have used a bit of Stretchercise to ease my anxiety ahead of the Pumas Test, but in the end it all went pretty well. We won 67–19 and I can't remember us being overwhelmed by the bajada at all.

I got half an hour off the bench against France in Wellington — another comfortable win — before we moved into the critical part of the season: the Bledisloe Cup and Tri Nations.

The Bledisloe didn't go well. We lost in Dunedin, so the cup was staying in Australia no matter what happened in Sydney, but pride was at stake, and we had a great chance to win that game. We were leading by four points as we went into the final minute. I was on for Hoefty and could only look on as Stephen Larkham threw an inside pass to Toutai Kefu off a strike move from a lineout, Ron Cribb missed a regulation tackle and the big loose forward crashed over. The Wallabies went nuts, which was fair enough.

We weren't a great team, and I wasn't a great player. I didn't feel comfortable at that level, but nor did I feel overawed. I knew I had to get more technically aware and develop some consistency, but I was looking forward to using that All Black experience as a launching pad.

I should be so lucky.

I barely played for Otago in the NPC that followed. The campaign had already started and Laurie Mains preferred Kees at tighthead. It never felt like a competition. I liked the bloke — he was a 'Bad News' Aucklander and he and Hoefty used to play off each other and had this real exaggerated bro thing going on, even though they came from vastly different backgrounds. I was given a bit of time at loosehead prop but I could never get comfortable on that side of the scrum. I was average and even though we made the final — losing to Steve Hansen's Canterbury — it felt like a bit of a wasted campaign for me.

In the meantime, Smithy had started having doubts after a couple of difficult years in charge of the All Blacks. Those doubts were echoed by the board of New Zealand Rugby and he was out of a job and John Mitchell, backed by Robbie Deans, was in.

Given my struggles to have any impact in the NPC, and a bad lack of rhythm when I did play, I could see the writing on the wall for the end-of-year tour.

Sure enough, Mitchell didn't pick me. Kees and Yoda were preferred at tighthead, while Greg Feek and Dave Hewett, both from Canterbury, were the other props. It was my first really serious setback as a senior player, but my personal disappointment was eased by the selection of my old King's mate Tom Willis, who even captained the non-Test games on tour. I was really happy for him. I'd envisaged playing with him for 10 years, but it never worked out. He had to leave Dunedin for opportunities at Waikato and the Chiefs and we never did play for the All Blacks together.

If I thought I was going to ease into 2002, then I didn't see Laurie coming, who was brought in to replace Peter Sloane as coach of the Highlanders. In a way, that period shaped me for the rest of my career, because it was where I learned that you can't die in training: that no matter how physically spent you thought you were, there's this motor in your heart that will just keep pumping.

The training was tough. It made me mentally tough. These days, some of the stuff Laurie did at training wouldn't wash. The modern player would just say: 'No. I'm not doing any more 150-metre sprints. It's getting stupid.' But we hadn't reached that point in rugby's player-power evolution. It was not like it was training without purpose. Laurie wanted us to be the fittest and strongest team and we were there, or thereabouts. We just lacked a bit of finesse to get us past the Crusaders in that year's final.

Kees had shifted back home to Auckland and the Blues, so I moved up Laurie's pecking order. Despite making the final in his first year, Laurie's two-year stint in charge of the Highlanders was a period of turmoil. I didn't mind the bloke — he was a King's and Southern man himself, so I felt some kinship there — but guys like Anton and Simon Maling chafed at his autocratic style.

Laurie wasn't the warmest bloke you were going to meet, but he knew rugby and he could definitely coach. Yes, he was probably a man out of his time when he came back to the Highlanders after a stint in South Africa, but if you could put aside your feelings about him as a person, he did some good things. We were moving into an era, however, when players expected to be able to have conversations with their coach, not just be told what to do and when, even when away from the field.

He was demanding from a training point of view and he definitely had two sides to his personality. There was the ruthless side. He wasn't the sort of guy you wanted to cross or upset because he held grudges. But at the same time, I never recall him yelling and screaming like a typical French coach, for example. Laurie preferred mind games, approaching you during a training drill and saying: 'Carl, are you sure you're doing the right thing there?'

It was never actually a question. It was code for, 'Sort your shit out.'

Touring with Laurie was never relaxing. He'd call the most unnecessary meetings, sometimes because he 'sensed a looseness' in the squad or because someone had drawn attention to an article in a local paper that pinpointed our weaknesses. I wouldn't have been surprised if he'd used his old contacts there and planted the story himself. There was one I recall that had printed a combined best 15 of us and the South African team we were playing. It had hardly any Highlanders in it. Laurie made a big deal of that, and I guess he thought that might galvanise the team but the guys, especially the more cerebral ones like Anton, didn't want that kind of pop psychology. They just wanted tactics and strategy.

Laurie hated doors slamming and he hated people laughing. But of all the things he hated, and Laurie hated a lot of things, the thing he hated most was cheese. When it came to the effect it had on rugby performance, Laurie thought cheese was food concocted by the Devil himself.

In the week before a game against the Stormers in Cape Town, we went out to an Italian restaurant as a treat, because we'd won the week before. An otherwise pleasant evening was ruined by Taine Randell ordering the quattro formaggi pizza and Laurie laying into the team doctor because of it. The doctor was giving it back to Laurie, telling him to stop treating people like little kids. It was a real mood killer, and even though we beat the Stormers by a point and outplayed them physically, I wouldn't mind betting all that Laurie could think about as it unfolded was the gorgonzola fermenting in Taine's gut.

I didn't play any of the June Tests or the Bledisloe Cup and Tri Nations matches, but I did get a call-up for the end-of-year tour. It was a bit of a controversial tour, with a number of guys picked who didn't go on to have long careers. There was talk of the jersey being sullied, or cheapened, which was a bit rough on newer players like myself.

It wasn't a great tour for me. It was my first time under Mitchell and Deans and that was a bit of an eye-opener. At one point, we were sitting down to a visual presentation and one of the slides was this bridge coming out of New Zealand and joining Australia and that was our 'journey' to the World Cup. There was a fair bit of cynicism among the guys in the team. We'd talk about this journey in pretty interesting terms, usually with a swear word in front of it, which I don't think was Mitchell's intention when he created the concept.

I didn't feature much on tour. I came on for a couple of minutes in the 20–20 draw against France as a yellow card replacement for Kees, and I was on the bench against England, a Test we lost when Ben Blair was bundled out in the corner with time nearly up, but I never got on the field. I did start against Wales alongside Keven Mealamu and Tony Woodcock, the first Test we played together. We won easily enough, but the scrums were a hell of a mess and Gethin Jenkins got the better of me. There were a couple of particularly bad ones just prior to me being replaced by Kees. As I trudged off, I met the eye of Andrew Hore on the bench — he was an unused and dispirited sub — and I can't remember whether it was him or me, but one of us said: 'Oh well, that looks like our All Black careers finished.'

The tour had a funny feel to it and I came back home feeling pretty deflated by the experience and not at all confident that Mitchell and Deans rated me. In fact, I was pretty sure they didn't. I felt like I had blown my only opportunity in the game against Wales. You'd never have believed the relationship I'd forge a few years later with Kevvie and Woody. The number of scrums Woody and I would put down against each other in training over the next five years would be impossible to count. We have this running joke. When we see each other, we'll start singing that Barbra Streisand song: *'Memories / all alone in the moonlight,'* as we recall those days.

The next year, 2003, was a bit of a write-off. Gordie Hunter died, which was bloody upsetting and things blew up at the Highlanders, which was sadly predictable and maybe unavoidable. By the time the season play-offs rolled around, it was clear Laurie Mains couldn't continue beyond 2003, because he wouldn't have had many players left. All the same, the issue had to be handled with care and sensitivity. A players' meeting was called in the week before our final round-robin match (amazingly, if we'd beaten the Reds, we'd still have had a chance of making the semi-finals). Players' Association boss Rob Nichol flew down for the meeting and Alex McKenzie of New Zealand Rugby also attended. A document was shared among the attendees that outlined our concerns and which we were to sign off on before presenting it to Otago and Highlanders' management.

In his book, Anton wrote of my input to the meeting: 'Everyone appeared in full agreement with what was being said in an open forum where some of the tension was eased by Carl Hayman turning up with two dozen Speight's and saying gruffly that "he didn't want anyone to get thirsty".'

That's how I tended to respond to tension: with a joke or a beer.

Laurie would have had the chance to retire with some dignity had it not been for Otago CEO John Hornbrook, who really didn't seem to have much time for him. We had all agreed that the contents of the document — letter, call it what you will — would remain confidential, but he went on the record saying the players were living in a climate of fear and the document was 'like a letter from Dachau'. Fuck me! You can imagine how Laurie reacted to that! It all got really ugly, and left a pretty sour taste in my mouth. You can say what you like about the guy, but Laurie had done a lot for rugby in the region. He deserved a more dignified exit than he was allowed.

Laurie wasn't the only one who suffered. Some of the players, particularly Anton, were seen as troublemakers. I don't know if that particular shitfight had any bearing on World Cup selection but Anton, who also didn't have a lot of time for Mitchell and Deans, wasn't selected and neither was I. Mind you, my non-selection was far easier to justify, given I had never really featured under that regime. There had been training camps leading up to the World Cup and Deacon Manu, who I had assumed sat below me in the pecking order, had been invited and I hadn't, so the writing was being written in broad strokes on the wall. As a result, I wasn't involved in the Tri Nations that year, either, not even in the wider squad.

It might not sound like it given what happened at the Highlanders, but I'm not a guy who bags coaches. I tend to get on with it, no matter who is in charge. But I have to admit I was getting frustrated by Mitchell. I got some feedback from him, and although the specifics of it are gone from my memory now, I remember at the time thinking it was pretty average, dismissive and paint-by-numbers stuff. I didn't have as much to do with Deans, but I know the Crusaders guys rated him highly, the rest less so. I felt a bit lost by the end of the year. I saw myself as having most of the physical and technical attributes needed in a modern prop, but I wasn't getting the consistency of selection or even opportunities.

When Ted and Shag came in the following year, they made it obvious from the start that they believed in me and that was all I needed.

I could start to look mid- to long-term. I didn't have to worry about my next bad scrum being my last.

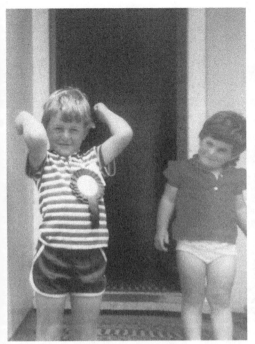

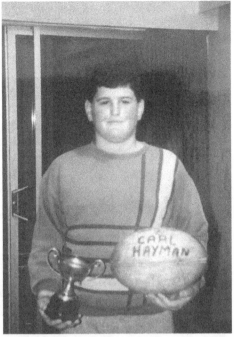

Me and my sister Stacey after coming second at the Ōpunake beach carnival Mr Muscle competition, 1985. Ōpunake is where I was born and raised – a small farming community on the southwest coast of Taranaki in New Zealand's North Island.

An award after playing for Ōpunake. The ball is my first ever rugby ball. I still have it to this day.

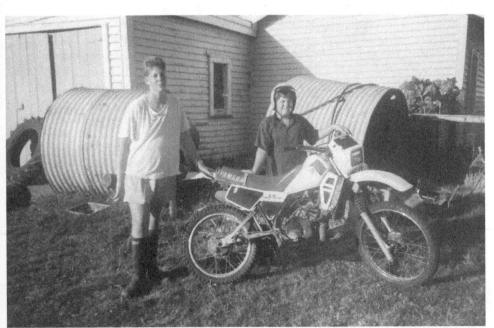

Me and my uncle Paul O'Rorke after a session on the YZ 125. I loved growing up on a farm. I can't imagine a better place to be a kid. You had space – literally – to grow and develop a type of self-reliance that is hard to replicate in an urban environment.

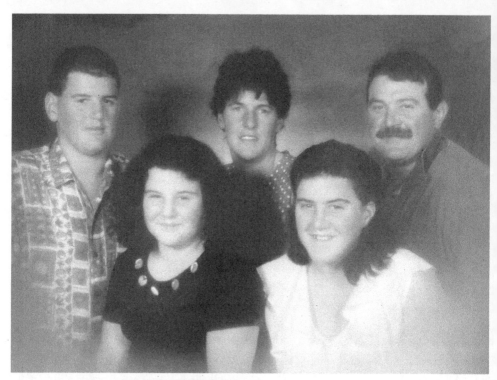

Above: Mum, Dad, and my sisters Stacey and Rebecca, circa 1993. Mum's family, the O'Rorkes, are a multi-generational Ōpunake family. Growing up in a rural environment, I watched Mum and Dad work bloody hard. Much of my work ethic I put down to their influence. Soon after this we moved to Otago. Many people assume I spent all my young life in Otago, because they associate me with Otago rugby teams. But if you ask me, I'll say I'm Taranaki through and through.

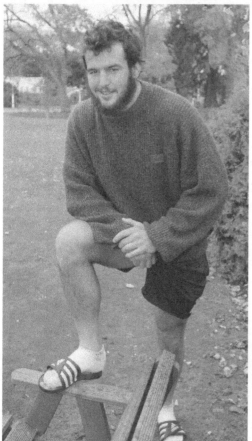

Left: A 'fresh-faced' Southern Man in Dunedin at the media press call in May 2001 after it was announced I had been selected for the All Blacks. In hindsight, I probably should have thrown a pair of jeans on! *Ross Land/Getty Images*

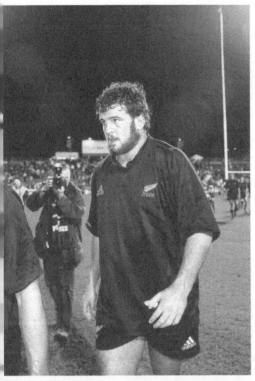

'All Black #1000'. A 21-year-old All Black prop, my first of 46 appearances for the All Blacks. North Harbour Stadium, Auckland, 16 June 2001. *www.photosport.nz*

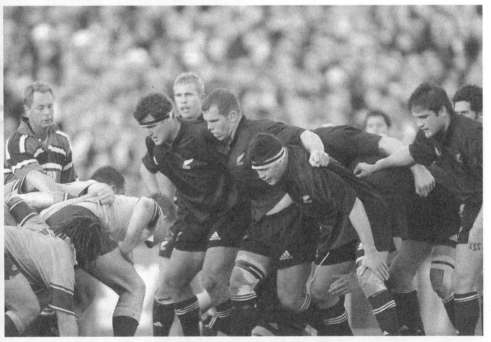

The front row packing down against the Wallabies, with Anton Oliver (middle) and Carl Hoeft to my right. The match was at Carisbrook — also known as the House of Pain. The Wallabies were world champions and had players like Joe Roff, Stephen Larkham, Matthew Burke. They were also captained by John Eales and coached by Eddie Jones. Even though Jonah Lomu opened the scoring, we lost the game 23–15 and in the process lost the Bledisloe Cup. A tough year to be an All Blacks rookie! Dunedin, 11 August 2001. *Sandra Teddy/www.photosport.nz*

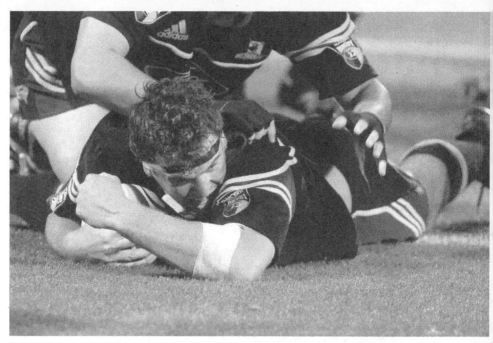

If I thought I was going to ease into 2002, then I didn't see Laurie Mains coming, brought in as coach of the Highlanders. In a way, that period shaped me for the rest of my career, because it was where I learned that you can't die in training: that no matter how physically spent you thought you were, there's this motor in your heart that will just keep pumping. March 2002, Highlanders v Cats. *Simon Baker/Getty Images*

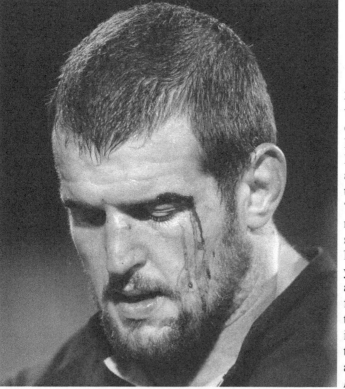

2003 was a bit of a write-off. I had fallen out of favour with the All Blacks coaches Robbie Deans and John Mitchell and wasn't selected for the Rugby World Cup. There was also a big rift in Otago between some of the players and Laurie Mains. It was a year to forget. When Ted and Shag came in the following year to coach the All Blacks, they made it obvious from the start that they believed in me and that was all I needed. *Ross Land/Getty Images*

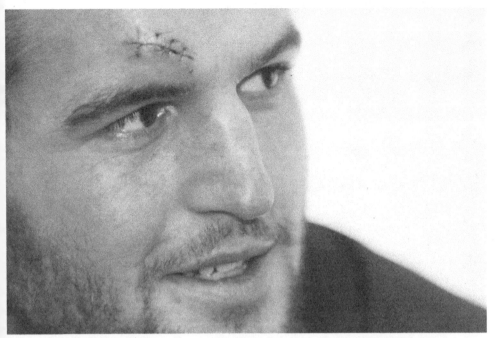

Stitches on my forehead from wounds received during the test match against England at Carisbrook, 15 June 2004. I didn't suffer too many serious injuries during my long career, but I played close to 450 games of first-class rugby, so my brain was exposed to thousands of head knocks. *Ross Land/Getty Images*

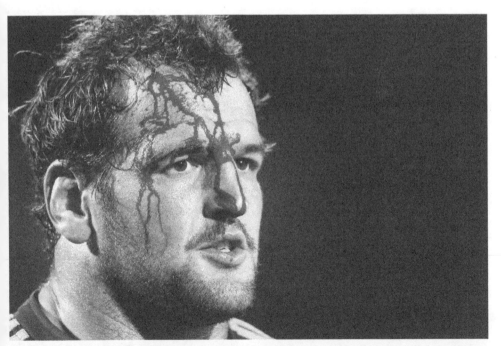

Super 12, playing the Reds in Brisbane, 2005. It wasn't uncommon to 'see red' throughout my career. In the early days especially I felt I was 10-foot tall and bulletproof. Later, when I brought down the curtain on my career, I took immense pride in the fact that I had literally played through pain to set up my family's future. *Jonathan Wood/Getty Images*

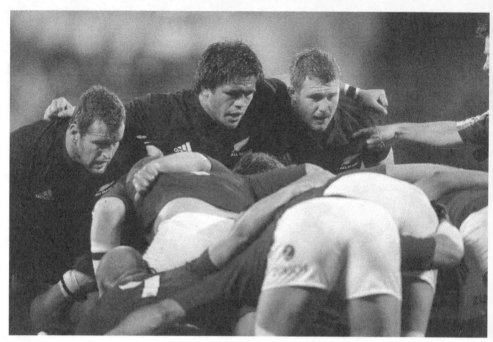

Packing down in the scrum with Keven Mealamu and Tony Woodcock against the Lions in 2005, Jade Stadium, Christchurch. Playing against the Lions was a once-in-a-lifetime event. *Ross Land/Getty Images*

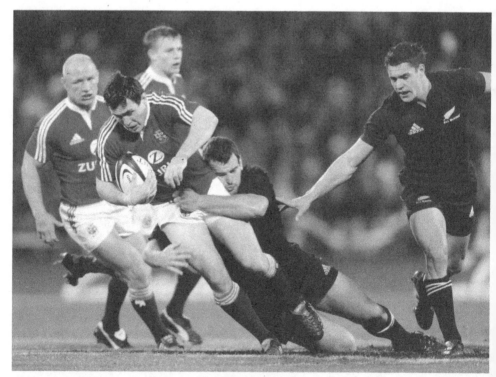

Tackling Stephen Jones in the first test against the British and Irish Lions, Jade Stadium, Christchurch. We would eventually win the series 3–0. *David Davies/Getty Images*

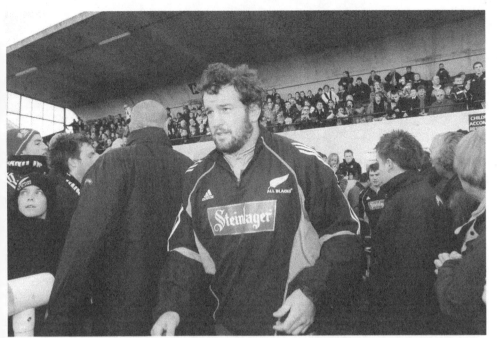

Drinking on tours was still a big part of All Blacks culture in 2005. It was a hangover from the amateur days, when tours were not just a chance to play footy, but also to take part in a giant boys' trip. It was a cherished part of touring life. This photo was taken on the Grand Slam tour of the UK and Ireland. We completed the Grand Slam that year, beating Wales, Ireland, England and Scotland in the month of November. The tour would also become known for boozy hijinks, after a few of the boys hit the town in Cardiff after a Saturday training. *Sportsbeat Images*

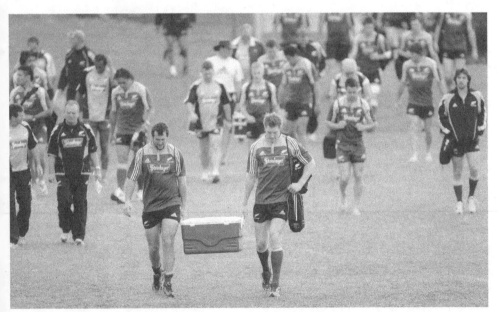

All Blacks training in Durban, South Africa. Although it remained, it was only once Ted Henry came in at the All Blacks in 2004 that I really experienced any moderation of the drinking culture embedded in the team. South Africa, August 2005. *Ross Land/Getty Images*

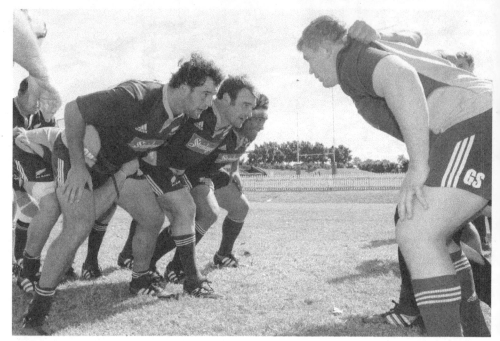

My fate at tighthead prop was sealed when I was 15 years old. It felt right from the first time I hit a scrum machine. The tighthead packs down with his head between those of the opposing hooker and loosehead. Both his ears are jammed up against opposing players: his head is 'tight'. All Blacks training session, July 2006. *Hannah Johnston/Photosport*

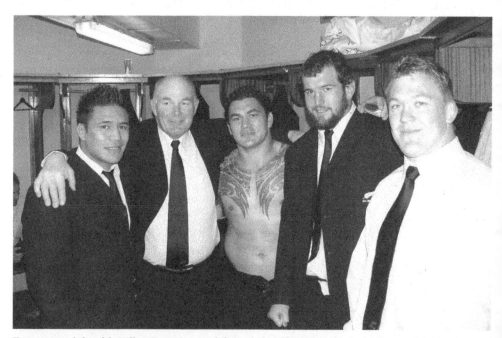

Front row club with Mike Cron (second from left). There's nobody in the world who knows as much about scrums as Mike Cron, who has worked with World Cup-winning All Blacks and Black Ferns teams. He's got a great saying about the difference between a loosehead and a tighthead prop: 'A loosehead pisses with the wind at his back, a tighthead pisses into the wind.'

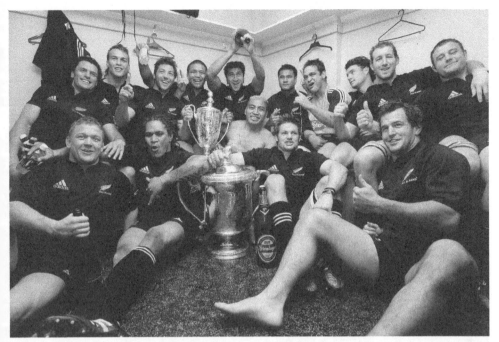

In the changing room after winning the Bledisloe Cup against Australia at Eden Park in 2006. During the match I suffered a head clash with Wycliffe Palu, which left me concussed and ataxic. I have no recollection of the night that followed. *Phil Walter/Getty Images*

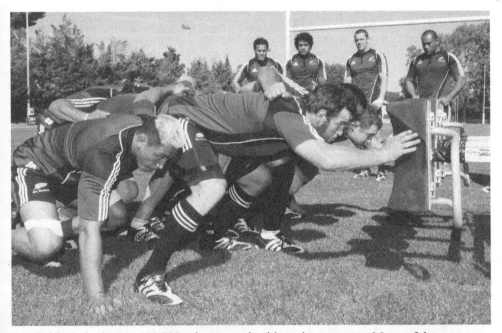

I probably took close to 150,000 sub-concussive blows in my career. Many of these were simply the sort of head-rattlers you get from putting down scrum after scrum against a machine. September 2007. *Ross Land/Getty Images*

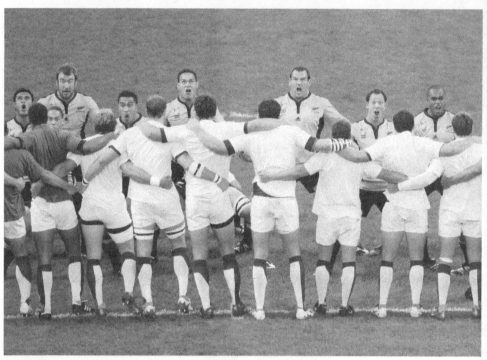

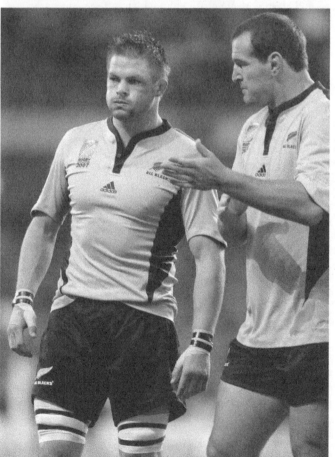

Above: Our haka before taking on France in the 2007 quarter final in Cardiff. We were supremely confident going into the 2007 world cup. We'd only experienced three defeats in the previous three seasons. *Laurence Griffiths/Getty Images*

Left: Cardiff, 2007. 'Game Plan Two' Those three words are all you need to say to trigger a flood of memories. *Marc Weakley/ Photosport*

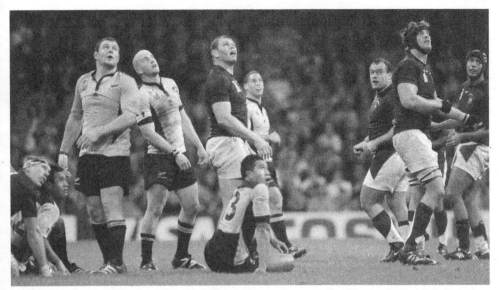

Both teams look towards the posts as Luke McAlister attempts a desperate drop-goal on the road to losing the game 20–18. *Andrew Cornaga/Photosport*

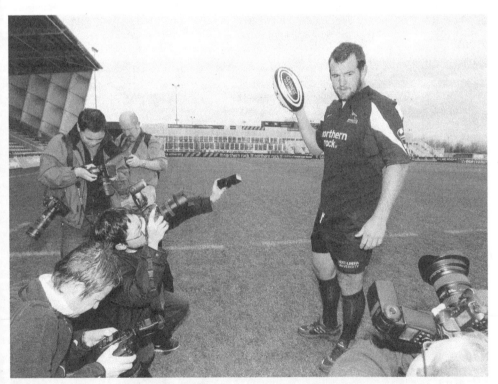

'Million-dollar man', November 2007. The year had been a weird one, what with the ill-fated World Cup campaign and the death of my grandfather. The latter had put the former into perspective. I knew that my career was short and that life was worth living. *Owen Humphries/Getty Images*

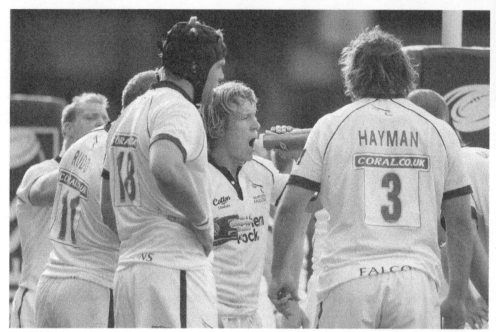

When I got to Newcastle, I noticed an immediate change in the drinking culture. We had Jonny Wilkinson and Toby Flood, who didn't drink at all, and there were no court sessions or any real team bonding over alcohol like I was used to from my days with Otago and the All Blacks. 21 September 2008. *David Rogers/Getty Images*

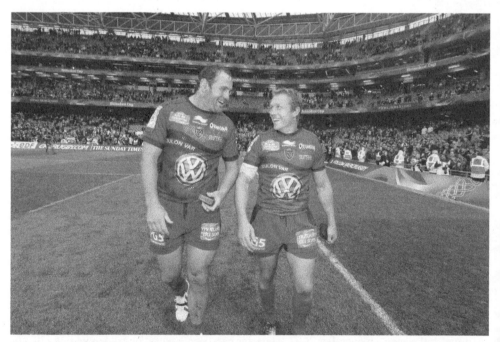

Celebrating with Johnny after our victory at the end of the Heineken Cup final against ASM Clermont Auvergne at Aviva Stadium in Dublin, 2013. Unfortunately, it was at Toulon where my drinking started to become problematic. Well, I'll rephrase that: it was already problematic, but it was there where it started to have ramifications beyond my own personal health. *David Rogers/Getty Images*

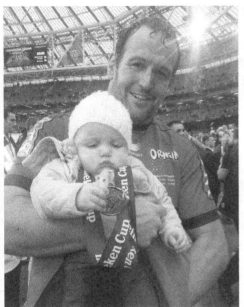

Winning in Europe was a wonderful feeling. We would win three Heineken Cups in a row, and a Top 14 title in the 2013–14 season. They were my glory days but it was also when my cognitive decline started to become apparent. I just didn't recognise it at the time.

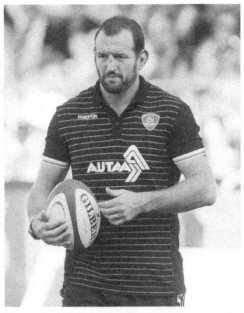

September 2016, coaching Pau in the French Top 14 match against Bayonne. If there was a lesson I learned during my time in the little French town of Pau, it's that things can always get worse. It wasn't just a matter of getting angry and irritable. At team meetings, I found myself welling up when talking – literally holding back tears.

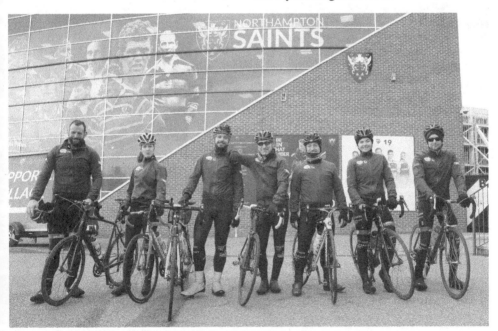

The Great Rugby Cycle 2019 in support of Doddie Weir's Foundation, Northampton, 13 March. This is prior to our departure from Franklin's Gardens on the next stage of their trip from John O'Groats to Land's End. *David Rogers/Getty Images*

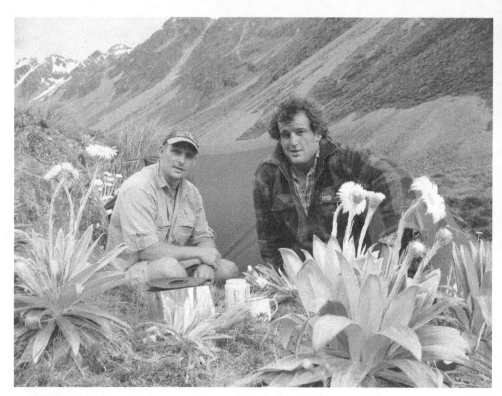

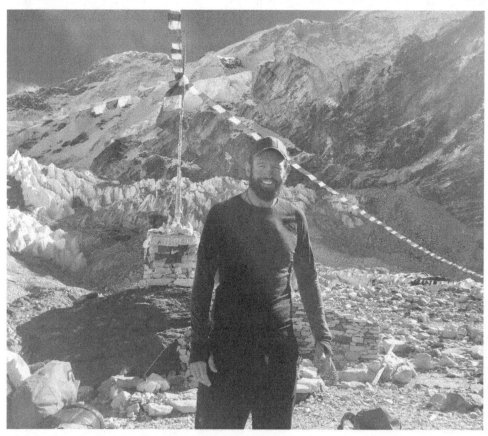

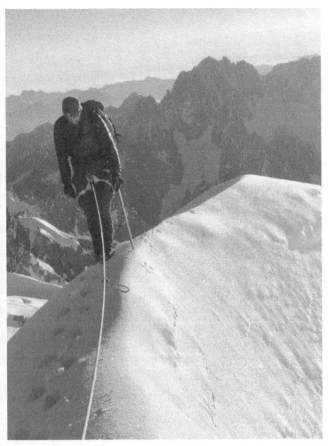

Whether it's completing Ironman, hunting in the New Zealand back country or climbing mountains in the French Alps or the Himalayas, I have always been drawn to the outdoors. It's where I find the most happiness. Over the past few years, I've noticed a considerable decline, not just in my cognition, but also in my energy levels. But exercise remains one of the best things I can do manage my symptoms.

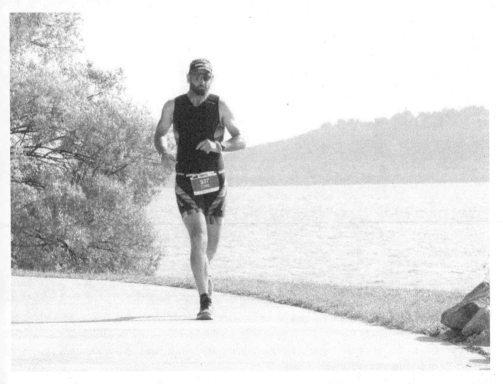

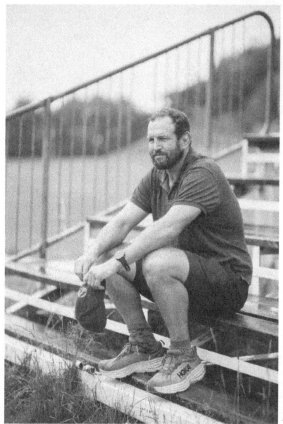

I struggle with the concept of 'the future'. It's been a weight on my mind, and when I think too much about it, I get scared. Through the course of my long rugby career – a career I can look back on with pride – I was living life with the accelerator pressed down hard. I played hard, I trained hard, I partied hard. To some extent, that continued post-career. I was always conscious of the next goal, whether it was completing an Ironman, or climbing mountains. *Matt Quérée*

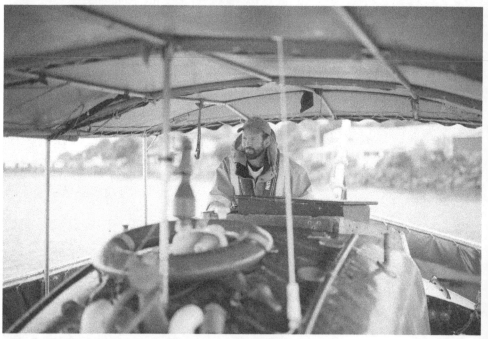

February 2023. My boat, *Rescue III*, has provided a frighteningly apt metaphor for where I am in my life at the moment. I might not have her good looks, but I'm dinged up, requiring a bit more work than I can imagine, but I think I'm worth persevering with. *Matt Quérée*

7

MAKALU, 2019, HEAD IN THE CLOUDS

AN EXCERPT FROM MY diary:

Day 1. Kathmandu to Lukla — Mera Lodge, 3500m

I need to start with the reasoning behind this trip. I have always been drawn to the outdoors and the mountains. From living next to Mt Taranaki as a kid or hitting the hills around Dunedin, outdoor life is where I find the most happiness. I am setting off on this expedition to Makalu to realign myself with the environment that I love, but also to find out more about myself. One great

thing about Nepal is the spiritual power of the country.
Buddhism has been a way of life here for many centuries.
I hope to learn and grow the spiritual side of me, which
has slowly developed over the last few years. Also, this
is a huge physical challenge. I want to test my limits
and see how I react and, mentally, what my response
is to various situations that will present themselves on
the mountain. I will aim to keep a diary so that maybe
Sophie, Taylor or Charles might want to follow this path
[one day], or at least read about the expedition.

Today was a long one, with a wake-up call at 5.15 am
for our 7.30 flight. Travelling to the airport, I was
nervous about the weight we had to take to Lukla. Our
15 kg limit was not going to cut it and we had huge
carry-on bags. Mine was a 60l mountain pack! During
the week we had a benediction and it must have worked
as after a lot of discussion we were all able to board, but
our big bags would be on a later flight.

Lukla is well known for being a dangerous airport
and you can see why. The airport is situated in the valley
but the runway finished into the hillside meaning no
aborted landings and normally unpredictable winds.
Once we landed, we collected our bags and [had] about
3 hours walking to Mera Lodge (3500m), a quiet little
lodge and it's early season here so not a lot of people.
Being early season, there were a few washed out bridges

and we reconstructed one and got wet feet on the other. Rain is frequent throughout early September until the end of the monsoon.

Have been thinking a lot about Sophie, Taylor and Charlie today. Am missing those little guys and I'm really looking forward to getting home in November. One hell of an adventure ahead of us. Excited.

* * *

Every now and then you meet somebody in your life who is the right person for the right time. I'm lucky to have met a few, from Eoin Willis at King's High, the man who moved me from lock to prop, to Kiko, of course. But there's another bloke who has played a more pivotal role in my life than he probably realises — a French climber and adventurer by the name of Franck Candelier.

I met Franck when walking the famous GR20 in Corsica, which runs diagonally across the island from Calenzana in the northwest to Conca in the southwest, as part of a charity event for Toulon. Ex-England lock Simon Shaw was part of the group, and we completed the 180 kilometres in a little more than six days. We lost toenails and our feet were basically giant blisters, but we raised 35,000 euros for sick children, so it was worth the mangled feet. Franck was using the GR20 to train for a Himalayan expedition, so I started hanging around with him at the back of the pack, listening to him talk about his trips to Nepal and trying out my pidgin French on him.

Franck was living in Ajaccio, the birthplace of Napoleon Bonaparte and very close to where we had enjoyed a pre-World Cup camp in 2007, but his big heart always resided in Nepal. I had never expressed much of an interest in alpinism, though I enjoyed telling Franck about hunting for tahr in the mountains above Tekapo. It was during these chats that Franck, who was training for a climb of Manaslu, the eighth highest peak in the world, planted the seed for me to join him one day on an expedition in Nepal.

Francky loves the mountains. This man with a gentle disposition and warm smile has been going back and forth to Nepal for more than 20 years. Even today, not a year goes by without a new Nepalese entry in his passport. His visits are always more about exploration than expedition. When he's not hiking in remote areas, he spends time with his many Nepalese friends, helping them improve living conditions in their villages.

He's just a guy you want to spend time with. He has a discretion and humility that puts you at ease and just being around him is enough to soak up his experiences and feel the echo of his passion for the mountains and outdoors.

In 2015, almost as a present to myself for retiring from rugby in one piece — or so I thought at the time — I flew to

Nepal to walk the Annapurna Circuit. In terms of mountain climbing, the Annapurna, while at high altitude, is the Nepalese version of the Tongariro Crossing or the Milford Track. It is a place of stunning beauty, but there's no technical climbing. There was something intensely spiritual about it, though, and it had been a long time since I had been at such peace with myself.

I wasn't at such peace with myself or the world in general when Franck contacted me to say he was taking an expedition to Makalu, at 8451 metres, the fifth highest peak in the world.

To help prepare, I ended up climbing Mt Blanc (4809 metres) with him a couple of times. We did it in a day once — caught the train from St Gervais to the first hut to start the ascent, got there, climbed it and tried to get down in time to catch the last train back. We just missed it. It's not an overly technical climb, but the first bit is a rock scramble and there's one section called the couloir de la mort, loosely translating as 'death row', where you're exposed to the danger of falling rocks. Obviously, I lived to tell the tale, but it was good preparation for trekking around in the high altitude of Nepal.

Day 4 Khote to Thanga.
As our walk followed the valley, the power of the river was certainly impressive. Twenty-five years ago, a lake burst up high and you can still see the height at which it

raced down the valleys. A small stop for lunch, as feeding the porters regularly is very important because without them, we won't be going anywhere. Even at 4000m you feel the effects of the altitude. Very occasionally gasping for air. After four days my head is starting to clear after dealing with some personal issues over the last while. I feel day by day I am thinking less about problems, trying to relax and let go a little.

I liked the idea of conquering one of the 14 peaks above 8000 metres. The idea grew on me, but rugby always got in the way. Franck and I kept in touch, though, and with me having lost my job at Pau, and with Nat and I separated and the kids living back in New Zealand, the time was right to start training and have a serious tilt at one.

I would be out of my comfort zone, both in the literal and figurative senses.

One of the attractions of this expedition was that most of the fun was getting to Makalu base camp. We were taking a route called the Three Cols Walk, which saw us scale three cols — a mountain pass between two peaks — all at an altitude above 5000 metres.

One of the cols had a sheer drop on the other side, which we had to abseil down. Abseiling does not come naturally to me, but I thought I'd done okay after inching my way down from crack to crack, toehold to toehold. Unclipped and taking in the new surroundings, I looked up to see a sherpa, a much older man than I, pretty much running down the cliff face, letting the rope run free.

Next time, maybe.

We had planned to take a crack at the Mera Peak summit on the way in, almost as a simulation for our later attempt on Makalu, but fate intervened.

Day 8: Mera Peak.

Slept poorly at 5700 m, quite normal. Was up at
1 am-ish and we left around 2 am for the summit...
Although the sky was clear, there was a good storm
system maybe 20–30 km to our left. The occasional
lightning flash would light up the horizon.

[Sherpa] Lakpa was at the lead of the group, weaving
his way through the crevasses, and there were plenty of
them. It was slow going but I was feeling strong despite
the quick rise in altitude over the last few days. The
temperature was very cold and I could feel my hands
starting to go. Trying everything to keep them warm
but to no avail. As the sun broke about 5 am, we had
an amazing silhouette of Everest, Lhotse, Cho Oyu and
Makalu. I looked in awe at what we would be climbing
in a few weeks. I was feeling good at this stage, but the
storm was now approaching. Also, Franck and Denis
have been struggling with the altitude. We decided

to turn around at 6200 m, 200 m from the summit. Although disappointing not to summit, Mera has served its purpose as a good training run… we were officially on our way to Makalu.

We would stop at small huts along the way to Makalu base camp. We'd sit around a fire, smoke would envelop you and suddenly someone would emerge with a steaming plate of potatoes. A bit of chilli, a bit of salt. That would be lunch.

Occasionally you get the opportunity to buy a can of Coke for 1000 rupees. At the time, the exchange rate was 123 rupees to one dollar, so at about $8 per can, the mark-up was pretty steep. But if you craved that instant sugar hit, you paid. There were no supermarkets on the route, so we were a captive market.

While I was in the Himalayas, I was determined to try to learn more about the Buddhist way of life. I sidled up to Purna, one of the porters, and asked him about some of their mantras. He taught me a few, but only one stuck: 'Om Tare Tuttare Ture Soha'. Sitting in a tent, legs crossed and feeling the pain in my hip, a legacy of my career, I repeated the chant over and over. I have no idea what it meant, but after a while I opened my eyes to see Purna had fallen asleep and the snow was falling, almost in slow motion, outside. I was having some kind of spiritual moment for sure. I made a point to get alongside Purna more before we climbed Makalu.

Days 19, 20, 21

Snow, rain and generally unpleasant weather has
hampered progress at base camp. Lines are fixed to
Camp 2, but… due to the placement of Camp 1 and
the steep snow wall to climb to Camp 2, it's safer to stay
here, at least till we get a few days clear weather. The
plan is to advance to Camp 2, re-descend then push
to Camp 3 and then back down, meaning a summit
attempt might be possible early October.

Been thinking a lot lately about the kids and what
the future holds for us all. Can't wait to see them again
and get down to Opunake!

Makalu is considered a more difficult ascent than Everest and
was, in fact, conquered later, by a French climbing expedition
in 1955. Sir Ed Hillary had been there in 1954, but illness in
his group meant they couldn't attempt the summit. Part of his
expedition involved searching for the abominable snowman,
or Yeti. Hillary reportedly visited a temple, where the monks
handed over three Yeti scalps — though they turned out to
be somewhat less exotic, belonging in a past life to two bears
and a goat. Still, it was a humbling experience to know I was
walking into places Sir Ed loved and where he was held in such
great affection.

* * *

Days 24, 25

Base camp. Snow has really hurt the prospect of us getting to the top. Lakpa and Paysanne are not able to get to Camp 3 at this point. As I write this, I'm in my tent with everything open watching the snow fall. A nice sight, but not for climbing! Lakpa and Paysanne have been waist deep in snow for the last two days trying to get to Camp 3. There are now serious doubts if we will get any higher than Camp 2 (6600 m), a real shame. I feel I have poured myself into this and am in good shape to push for the summit. Months of work, not to mention the financial commitment from everyone and sponsors, makes it hard. On a positive note, we have experienced an amazingly beautiful and challenging route in. Passing two cols over 6000 m and Mera Peak.

A few days of hope yet but the snow is still falling. It will be interesting to see how the other groups are going on other mountains, as the monsoon is normally finished 15 days ago and snow and poor conditions still persist.

And my final entry:

Day 27

Meanwhile, at Base Camp life has become very mundane. Cards have played a big part in the time-killing. Rummy. I'm not that great and often come in last… [The sherpas] leave tomorrow to have one last try at opening Camp 3. Nathan and Bill went to the local village and came back with rope for the fixed lines and a few supplies, notably a bottle of whiskey. Not sure when that will come out. Tomorrow it will be either green or red and there is not much we can do here. I am ready both physically and mentally. All my gear apart from two oxygen bottles is at Camp 2. I have been trying to eat as much as I can to keep my energy up, but I am starting to feel skinny.

We didn't make the summit. Although we had the mountain to ourselves for six weeks, it was too dangerous. It's a hellishly difficult, technical climb near the top. Just five of its first 16 attempts were successful and even recently the totals of 22 fatalities to 206 successful ascents of Makalu tell a story. That's basically one death for every 10 that attempt it, so if Franck and the team leaders said it was too dangerous, I wasn't going to waste my time arguing.

In terms of a life experience, it was pretty amazing. Despite the frustration experienced, with so much being out of your control — most notably the weather — I found it easy to get into a zen-like state.

Scaling an 8000-metre peak. That's still an itch I'd like to scratch.

8

CARDIFF, 2007, GAME PLAN TWO

GAME PLAN TWO.

Those three words are all you need to say to trigger a flood of memories. There's a few of us of a certain vintage who still keep in touch and when the All Blacks are struggling a bit, one of us will invariably send out a message along the lines of: 'Looks like they've gone to Game Plan Two.'

But I'm getting a bit ahead of myself. By now, you know the result of the 2007 RWC quarter-final, and you might even have come to terms with it. It's sometimes crazy to think as I write this: that match is 15 years in the past. A lot has happened since then, both in my life and the life of the All Blacks. Two victorious World Cup campaigns in 2011 and 2015 is no small thing — not that I'd play a part in either of them.

In the intervening years, a lot of blame has been apportioned for New Zealand's, to date, worst showing at a World Cup. There was 'rest and rotation', a well-meant but ultimately flawed idea that failed in its objective to keep players fresh for the tournament in France. There was playing people out of position, a mistake we swore we wouldn't make after Christian Cullen and Leon MacDonald, both fullbacks, were shoehorned into centre in 1999 and 2003 respectively. We ended up making it anyway. There was, of course, referee Wayne Barnes, the latitude given to France at the breakdown in that second half and that infamous forward pass.

Somehow, Game Plan Two has escaped scrutiny. By my reckoning, it hasn't warranted enough attention. That, for me, was where an otherwise good, well-thought-out campaign came crashing down. It was a lesson that sometimes even the best-run teams can overthink things; how even the strongest leadership groups can, through fatigue as much as anything else, fail to provide leadership when it's most needed.

That was a squad that you could say deserved better, but in the end, we got what we earned — a notoriously early exit in the quarter-final and a whole bunch of misery. Some found redemption four years later, but for many, like myself, it stayed with us a bit longer. Perhaps it was never truly rectified. Don't get me wrong: I don't sit on my boat reliving those 80 minutes, but there'll be times when I'm catching up with old teammates, or sometimes just at random moments, when those three words — Game Plan Two — will pop up. I can laugh about it now, but it took a while to see the funny side.

So how did a campaign that was meant to end with a glorious push into Paris end in Cardiff? Let's go back a few years.

* * *

My All Blacks career technically restarted in 2004, but in a sense, it was the beginning. I might have already had eight Tests under my belt, but six were off the bench and I'd struggled to impose myself on the thoughts of John Mitchell and Robbie Deans.

In 2004, Graham 'Ted' Henry, Steve 'Shag' Hansen and a rejuvenated Wayne Smith came on board with a bunch of fresh ideas.

They'd all had coaching experience overseas — Ted and Shag with Wales and Smithy at Northampton — and were keen to impart what they'd learned on their travels to this next chapter of All Blacks rugby.

Another thing that was not spoken about as much but which was apparent anyway, was that they wanted the All Blacks to project a better image off the field. Leading up to the 2003 World Cup in Australia, the All Blacks had been seen as arrogant and aloof. Mitchell and Deans had struggled to get on the same page as the media and there were even stories about big-money sponsors being snubbed by players and coaches at pre-planned events.

Speaking with the benefit of hindsight, the overseas experiences accrued by the new coaching and selection panel were a good thing. In New Zealand at that time, we tended to live in a rugby bubble, where we thought our way — the Kiwi way — was not just the best way, but the only way to play the game properly.

But rugby can be different. One of the beauties of the sport is that it is open to interpretation. Different styles can be effective depending on the strength of your personnel, the opposition, the conditions or even the referee.

We came to view '10-man rugby' as a dirty phrase but there is a place for forward-dominated rugby based around set piece and mauls. I guess a tighthead prop would say that, wouldn't he? Having coaches who had been exposed to what we might call the northern hemisphere style had the potential to make us so much more rounded. Depending on our squad limitations at any given time, having the ability to toggle between modes of playing could really be beneficial, as long as we prepared properly.

My biggest gripe about Super Rugby, particularly nowadays, is the teams are too similar. The New Zealand clubs all tend to play to a prescriptive style — essentially mimicking the All

Blacks — while the Australian teams play a style that is not too dissimilar from New Zealand's.

To jump ahead in time and digress a bit, New Zealand rugby is really going to miss the South African sides from a playing point of view, now that they have withdrawn from Super Rugby. Sure, they might not have provided the box-office appeal of a local derby, but in my day playing games against the likes of the Bulls were invaluable. They were a point of difference. You knew what was coming — a giant forward pack, a world-class lineout and halves that kicked all day — but it didn't necessarily mean you could stop it.

Back to 2007. The Henry era started well. We turned over the world champions, England, pretty easily in two Tests. We beat Argentina and the Pacific Islanders and won our home matches in the Tri Nations against South Africa and Australia. But it didn't take long before familiar cracks started appearing.

In our return match against Australia in Sydney, we got off to a great start and led handily. I even found myself running in open space a couple of times, which was a novel experience. We tightened up, however, to let them back in the game and then couldn't get over the line when we found ourselves trailing late in the match.

If that was frustrating — a slow-leak puncture — then the wheels really fell off in Johannesburg. We fell to a crushing 26–40 defeat at Ellis Park, the holiest cathedral in South

African rugby, but the loss was not as pivotal to the team's future direction as what happened afterwards.

Alcohol was still a big part of All Blacks culture. It was, literally, a hangover from the amateur days, when tours were not just a chance to play footy, but also to take part in a giant boys' trip. It was an accepted, even cherished, part of touring life.

After we were beaten by the Boks, we embarked on an epic court session with Carlos Spencer and Justin Marshall as judges. Court sessions were a common occurrence in those days, and were regarded as a fairly harmless way of letting off steam while we pored over the week that was and the various stuff-ups people had made along the way. The drinking was a big part of it, but what you normally did was get a keg in and your court session would last until it was finished. When you add up the players and staff who took part in the session, you're probably talking about 1 to 1.5 litres of beer each — not necessarily a healthy amount but not outrageously over the top either. Where it went wrong in Johannesburg was that top-shelf spirits were introduced into the fines. I'm not sure whose idea it was, and I guess it doesn't really matter. All that counts is that things went south pretty quickly from there. There were players and staff seriously twisted out of shape, and I remember one of the support staffers begging another not to leave him because he didn't know how he'd be able to get back to his room. The jury was definitely targeting the staff, but the players weren't immune. Simon Maling found himself in the toilets standing next to Sir Colin Meads, who was in South Africa, at the urinals. Simon was feeling the effects and like a scene from *From Dusk Till Dawn*, launched into a spew, some of which splattered over Pinetree's sleeve. Pinetree just brushed it off, looked at him and said: 'Good on you, boy.'

Watching all this carnage from the corner with a headmasterly look of scorn was Ted. I now understand how dangerous the normalisation of heavy drinking can be, but even back then I had enough awareness to realise that night was over the top and that there would be repercussions. No individual was to blame, and I don't think anyone had their cards marked, so to speak. The drinking was embedded into the culture of the team, not individuals, and every now and then it's going to go wrong. This was one of those nights.

Ted knew things had to change. I think Smithy was mortified, too. He'd tried to quietly instigate changes to the team's ethos, especially around drinking, when he was coach, to introduce a level of professionalism in that regard that he felt had been missing. I think he felt the standards had regressed again. On our return to New Zealand, meetings were held between management, captain Tana Umaga and Richie McCaw, who was being groomed for leadership. Certain edicts around socialising and how we presented ourselves were laid down. Out of that came the concept of the leadership group, which I, for my sins, would soon join. This was a big step in

the development of the All Blacks as a more professional —
in every sense of the word — high-performance unit, but it
did come with unintended consequences, which we'll address
soon.

One thing it didn't achieve was putting a full stop on boozy
hijinks. On our Grand Slam tour to the United Kingdom in
2005, a few of the boys hit the town in Cardiff after a Saturday
training. With a full week to go until the first Test of the
tour against Wales and a day off on Sunday, hitting a few of
the local hotspots didn't seem like such a bad idea. And it
wasn't, although believe it or not, I passed on the opportunity,
preferring to sleep off the last vestiges of jet lag. Most had a
decent night out before tucking themselves into bed in the early
hours. A few of the boys weren't keen on the night ending in
Cardiff, however, so Dan Carter, Piri Weepu, Aaron Mauger,
Jason Eaton, Jimmy Cowan and Leon MacDonald convinced a
cabbie to take them 240 kilometres to London, with the vague
idea of hooking up with former player Andrew Mehrtens at
the infamous antipodean Sunday club, The Church. Although
they had a box of beers for company on the trip, when the
sun started rising a level of sobriety started to take hold in a
couple of them and they pretty quickly realised they had made
a serious misjudgement. Sitting in a 24-hour McDonald's
waiting for The Church to open, they came to their senses and
quickly hightailed it to Paddington station to get a train back
to Wales. Sitting back smugly in Cardiff, word started to filter

through the rest of the team. I'm not sure if we were more appalled at the lack of judgement or impressed by the audacity of the plan, but either way we knew there would be a price to pay for the London Six.

We were summoned to a 'video' meeting, but instead Tana took the floor and reamed the players out. It was brutal and always means more coming from a teammate, a peer, than it does from a manager. That, in essence, is one of the main reasons for having a player-led leadership group: to set the tone in a relatable way, rather than just receiving instructions from coaches and managers. No one was spared, not even rookie Jason Eaton, who was reminded that he hadn't even played a Test yet, though that fact was relayed to him with a few more words starting with 'f'. DC — Dan Carter — comes across as a clean-cut guy, the golden boy of New Zealand rugby, but believe me, he's got a bit of mischief in him. He was fingered as the ringleader and was pretty sheepish that week. Whatever mental pressure that put him under, he responded against Wales at a heaving Millennium Stadium by having one of his greatest Tests, which pretty much summed up what a unique talent he was.

It turned out to be Tana's last tour. We won the Grand Slam, which was a fitting way to send out someone I had a lot of time for. He was also a world-class centre, having moved mid-career from the wing. He had everyone's respect and could bridge that gap between management and players pretty easily. His elevation from one of the boys to a captain to be respected and even a little bit feared was such a natural progression. I'll admit that I'd hoped the retirement talk was just that — talk — and that he would carry on. It came as a shock when he made it official, considering he still bossed the midfield, but nothing's forever in the game. It was his call and he'd been doing it for a while, so fair play to him. He was finding post-match recovery harder and when that's the case, the game stops becoming fun and feels like a 'proper' job. Quite apart from everything he'd achieved on the field, he'd been instrumental in turning the whole team culture around off it. It's one thing having coaches telling you what to do: it's another when you've got someone like Tana driving it.

I don't mean this as an indictment on Richie McCaw, who will go down as one of the greatest, if not *the* greatest, All Blacks ever, and had obvious leadership credentials from the get-go. But I've always thought if we could have stretched Tana's career out for two more years, even if it meant giving him extended breaks and limited training, we could have been looking at a very different scenario when we returned to Cardiff a couple of years later.

The England Test was by far the hardest of the tour, partly through our own doing. I thought we had the measure of them pretty much everywhere, except referee Alan Lewis's pocket. He dished out three yellow cards against us, which were nowhere near as common then as they are now, and none against England. At one stage, we had 13 men on, but we held on for the 23–19 win with some backs-to-the-wall defence in the final minutes. The reaction to the game was unintentionally hilarious. I wasn't involved, but I remember England winning in similar circumstances in Wellington in 2003 and the All Blacks were hammered by our press for failing to beat an undermanned England, whose performance was hailed as heroic. Were the roles reversed in 2005? You bet they weren't. England were again hailed as heroes by their media, while we were cynical offenders who would do anything to win by fair means or foul. I came to realise that when it came to the English press, you could never win and it was pointless trying. It was easier to sit back and laugh.

As a squad, at the conclusion of that tour, an easy win against Scotland at Murrayfield, it felt like we were heading in the right direction. We were almost playing two separate 15s. We were rotating players and keeping everybody fresh. The communication from management to the team was excellent and it felt like we had a clear plan for how we wanted to play the game. It was working.

The British teams struggled to stay with us, which was a continuation of how it had been earlier in the year when the British and Irish Lions toured. That was intense. The build-up seemed to have gone on for 12 months. The year before, a bunch of us had gathered at a park in London to film some ads for Adidas. The shoe company was sponsoring both teams and were keen to milk it for all it was worth, so a bunch of presumptive Lions players and All Blacks headed out to pretend to engage in a game of bullrush. What Adidas probably hadn't counted on was that many in the All Blacks contingent were coming straight from the famous (infamous?) Shepherd's Bush Walkabout, having completed the tour with a big win over the Barbarians at Twickenham the day before. Some of the guys, still feeling the effects of the grog, forgot they were mic'ed up and were inadvertently sharing stories of what had gone on the night before with the production team, who I'm not sure needed to hear them.

The Lions had been on everybody's radar, because we all knew it was a once-in-a-lifetime event. I wouldn't compare it to going to the Olympics, but it had that feel, where you spend so long building to a pinnacle and want everything to go right for just that one event. With England being the world champions, it meant even more to beat the Lions than usual.

My role in that series was limited. I played the first Test at Christchurch, which we won 21–3. It wasn't a great spectacle. It was freezing, the coldest game I've played in New Zealand. The rugby was dragged down to the conditions: it was very stop-start, and certainly not the rugby-fest that had been advertised — and all the talk in the post-match focused on a single incident. In the opening minutes of the game, Tana and Keven Mealamu had collaborated in a tackle on the Lions' captain and inspirational centre Brian O'Driscoll that had seen him upended and unceremoniously dumped to the turf, suffering a tour-ending shoulder injury in the process. As a team, we were just breathing a huge sigh of relief to have won an ugly game of footy after all the hype when the reaction to O'Driscoll's injury began to get a head of steam. It went above and beyond anything we'd ever seen before. You can understand why Brian was gutted, but the whole thing seemed wildly over the top. There was even a press conference re-enacting the incident like it was the Kennedy shooting.

I woke up the next morning feeling a lot more sore than normal. I was struggling to get around. I had gone into the game with a small cut on my foot, not much more than a scratch, but it was now tender and awkward to put any weight on. The following day, Monday, I woke feeling like crap and my foot had blown up to a grotesque size. You could see the infection snaking its way through the veins in my calf. It was pretty revolting. I ended up in hospital on a drip in Wellington for three days, being pumped full of antibiotics because I had septicaemia — bacterial blood poisoning, for the layman. It wasn't a pleasant time and obviously it meant I was going to miss at least the second Test at Wellington's Cake Tin.

The coaching staff described my absence to the media as a sore toe, which made it sound like I had an ingrown toenail or something. I thought they were underplaying the situation slightly, but it probably meant they didn't have to answer too many questions about it. I was a pretty sick boy and ended up watching DC's second Test masterclass from my hotel room with my uncle. He'd come down to Wellington and had a ticket for the Test but was happy to keep me company instead. Dan was sensational in the 48–18 win that night, outplaying Jonny Wilkinson and reminding all of us watching, including me, that if the tight five could do their core roles and get Carter front-foot ball in the right parts of the field, he would get the job done. He had not just the fundamental talent but also that x-factor that comes along once or twice in a generation. His kick-and-chase try down the right-hand touchline that night must be one of the greatest individual tries scored in a big Test match.

I played with great English flyhalf — that's first-five in proper rugby language — Jonny Wilkinson at Toulon, and I used to get asked all the time to compare him to DC. In many ways, your first five-eighth is like the quarterback of an American Football team. They can be so influential in what is happening. If they're having a bad day, the team tends to have a bad day. I find it hard to compare the two because they were both so different. It's like comparing Picasso and Steve Jobs — they're both geniuses, but they move in different circles. Jonny reminded me more of Richie McCaw, in that he had that relentless work ethic and desire to win, whereas DC had that x-factor that was impossible to quantify. Where they were similar is that although they were both comparatively small, they were brave and willing to put their bodies on the line.

Never underestimate the signal that sends to the rest of the team when your No. 10 — the glory boy — is happy to put himself in the hurt locker and do the unglamorous work. I've heard it said that if you're six points behind and needed a try, you'd want DC on your team, whereas if you're two behind, you'd want Jonny: it's an oversimplified way of looking at it, but I wouldn't necessarily disagree.

There was talk that I might play the third Test, but it was never realistic given that I'd been off my feet for a long time and had lost a bit of conditioning. I only started running halfway through the week of the third Test and I'd lost 4 kilograms in hospital, so I wasn't considered. Some people must have been wondering how a big, tough prop had managed to miss two Tests with a sore toe.

The tour did have one huge highlight for me, however, and that was playing in the Māori side that beat the Lions 19–13 in Hamilton. I qualified through my dad's side of the family. My iwi is Ngāti Apakura, which has marae from Pirongia south down to Te Kūiti along the Waipā River. I'm enjoying learning more about that side of my genealogy: my understanding is the tribe was virtually wiped out by Tainui, but in more recent times the surviving hapū have started to reorganise into a collective voice again. Anyway, the after-party the night of the match was a classic, pretty much the embodiment of every cliché you imagine when you try to picture such an event. We were staying at a motel and the guitars came out for a singalong in one of the rooms, while there were actual boil-ups happening in others.

The Lions Test wasn't my first experience with the Māori. That came in 2002 with a tour to Australia. I remember that tour mainly because we nearly won the Test in Perth, because we had a former CIB guy in the management team who could lip-read. He'd basically decoded the Wallabies' lineout and we stole about six off them, mainly through Taine Randell.

Heading into the 2007 season, World Cup year, I was fully entrenched in the leadership group, which had come about in response to what Ted and the manager Darren Shand considered to be a lack of off-field accountability in the squad. It was a sound concept, but as with anything new, it wasn't without its flaws, which I'd soon discover. I might have one or two names wrong, my memory isn't what it used to be, but I think the group at that stage consisted of Richie, Yoda, Jerry 'JC' Collins, Aaron Mauger, Chris Jack, Rodney So'oialo, Keven Mealamu, Anton Oliver and me.

We were gathered together in one of what had become an endless series of meetings to be told of the coaches' plans to rest us for a big chunk of the 2007 Super Rugby season. My memory of that meeting is that there was general consensus that the idea of missing some rugby was sound. It had obvious benefits. Well, general consensus apart from JC, that is. He might have played nice for the coaches, but behind the scenes he didn't get it. He called himself a 'soldier', and soldiers are more comfortable in battle. He had no real interest in handing his beloved Hurricanes jersey to somebody else, but decided it was better to play nice and not kick up a fuss about it.

That was JC. He had an insatiable desire to play footy. It's no secret that he had a tough upbringing in Porirua and for him the footy field was a place where he had the same advantages and disadvantages as everybody else. He was a tough, tough man, the sort of guy you hate playing against but love to have on your team. His tragic death after a motor accident in France in 2015, along with partner Alana, shook me to my core.

While there was agreement that a break worked into our season was a good idea, there were doubts as to whether the start of Super Rugby was the right time. This isn't hindsight talking, either: they were expressed at the time. What I struggled with was that the World Cup was in September, we'd finished the end-of-year tour in December and four weeks later we were back in camp getting super fit. It should have been balanced better. We should have been training in our own environment, but there was so much at stake. It was a complex balancing act, but we didn't get it right.

I don't want to put words in the coaches' mouths, but I got the feeling they saw it as the best they were going to get. Pulling us out of the Tri Nations, for example, was going to create issues with the broadcasters, who were paying top dollar to have the best available. If you're looking at it from a sports science perspective, ultimately what it led to was us being in peak physical form for the Tri Nations, not the World Cup.

On a personal level, that year got off to a bumpy start, and I can't blame anyone but myself for that.

The rugby season is long and challenging. You get to November and you're on a tour to Europe. I don't know how we've historically won so many games on those tours because you're absolutely fried. The coaches really earned their money because every player is so tired and you can slip into end-of-year party mode if you're not careful. It doesn't matter whether you're playing the Irish, Welsh, Scots, English, French or even the Italians: it's always touted as the biggest Test of their year. They all come at us hard and want to show to their public that even if they can't match us for skills, they can for physicality.

Once the tour is finished, we get December off, and before you know it, January rolls around again and you're back into the grind. It has a relentless quality to it that is just as hard to deal with mentally as it is physically.

Natalie, my partner at the time who would become my wife, was moving from Auckland to Dunedin for 12 months, so before she arrived, my mate Simon Hearsey and I decided to go up into Fiordland for a few days' hunting. Simon was a big hunting mate of mine. Oftentimes the Highlanders would play on a Friday night, and we'd leave in the truck straight afterwards to Lake Station in North Canterbury, to Tekapo or over to Fiordland. This particular trip we had planned was a little like the Holy Grail of hunting. We were looking for some freezer-fillers, but we'd also heard about this legendary rock overhang, a rock bivouac, that was near where we were planning to shoot. The spot was at the Edith Saddle, a day's walk in and a day's walk out once we had taken my 5.5-metre Stabicraft across Lake Te Anau and up the Glaisnock River.

To say I was looking forward to the trip was a bit of an understatement, so I was mortified to learn it clashed with my first week of training in Dunedin with Anton Oliver. We all had pre-season training programmes that were fairly strictly regimented. It was just me and Anton in Dunedin, so New Zealand Rugby pulled in Brendan 'Cheese' Timmins, a robust Highlanders lock whose son Sam is now a Tall Black, to oversee and monitor us.

Spending five or six days hunting deer, with long days of walking up hills with heavy packs, was, I thought, as good as any fitness regime that could be cooked up in the gym. In all seriousness, I attribute the fact that I rarely got injured and avoided the usual ankle and knee complaints to my outdoor life. If you're forever negotiating tree roots and clambering up and down rocky shelves, your knees and ankles naturally get very strong.

I saw the conditioning window in 2007 as a time for, yes, conditioning, but also to have some mental time away. I don't think I had the confidence or wherewithal to communicate this with the coaching staff, but I was stubborn enough to stick to my guns. I'd do it my way. I just wouldn't tell anybody about it. At that stage of my life, I wasn't a good communicator. I rang Cheese and told him my plans and he was pretty much: 'thanks for letting me know'. He didn't have any real authority over me, so he was a soft mark. It was when he took it up the chain that all hell started to break loose and my phone was running red hot. It started to peak when I was piloting my boat up the northern arm of Lake Te Anau. Darren Shand, the manager, seemed pretty keen to reach me, so Simon and I made the executive decision to accidentally drop my phone off the side of the boat. If anyone fancies a swim, there's a perfectly good Nokia 3310 resting on the bottom of Lake Te Anau. I remained without a cellphone for the next 10 months or so and missed out on a few things as a result, but I also saved myself a bit of stress.

The outdoors was baked into me from a young age. As a kid, my mates and I used to camp a lot. Dad would get us to load the four-wheeler and we'd go and camp down by the creek at the back of the farm, no parents. I had a Rambo knife I'd been given for Christmas and a pack of Sizzlers. That's all we needed. So hunting was never about bloodlust for me. It was about getting out into the backcountry with good company and cooking up some pretty average feeds in rudimentary huts. Every now and then we surprised ourselves with our culinary prowess. I made a bread-and-butter pudding one trip out of a loaf of bread, some chocolate and a tin of condensed milk. That kept the boys going for a week. There's something really grounding about backcountry hunting. You come back to civilisation and have a shower and it's the greatest high you can have. You come back and walk into a supermarket and can choose what you want to eat. It's amazing. Everybody should do it once.

It was also a way of turning off the professional sport tap for a while. As I said, the rugby season can feel endless, with games and tournaments seeming to roll into each other. Despite the harsh terrain and hours on your feet, I would always come back from these hunting trips feeling fresher.

For a country kid, even Dunedin felt like a big city, so every now and then I felt an overwhelming urge to get out of town and into the country. So I did, and almost got myself in real trouble on the Edith Saddle when tripping and sliding 20 metres down a rock ledge. I had time to consider sticking my leg out, but thought the chances of a broken tibia were too high, so I stopped myself with my arse. My tailbone ran into a rock, and I stopped, all right. I had massive bruising around my coccyx and when I got back into the gym, it hurt like hell to do squats, but decided it was best to keep that injury and the reasons behind it to myself.

Even as I relished traipsing about in the bush, I felt bad that in the first week of what promised to be a huge year, Anton was basically training on his own. But you know what else: it was totally worth it. We bagged a 12-pointer red deer that had got its way into the wapiti block. You don't want red deer mixing with wapiti because they interbreed and weaken the wapiti strain. So while Shandy might not have been impressed, I was doing my part for the genetic integrity of the local fauna.

When I got back, I trained very, very hard. Anton didn't seem to take my absence to heart and didn't hold it against me. In some ways we're very different but in others we're cut from the same cloth. We both had interests outside of rugby and didn't necessarily want to be defined by the sport we were lucky enough to be pretty good at. If I could be accused of not thinking enough, at times Anton could overthink things. He immersed himself in everything he did and was always inquisitive. I could never work out whether he was a coach's dream or a nightmare because he was never afraid to challenge conventional wisdom. He'd been fairly unimpressed with the culture of the All Blacks when he was a youngster trying to establish himself, and he didn't believe in the idea that players should be seen and not heard. It's no secret that he struggled with Laurie Mains. Those two were like oil and water, and while I might not agree with the way Laurie's departure was handled, I understand that Anton was just trying to create the best Highlanders environment.

We really pushed each other hard. Anton was so motivated. He saw this as his last hurrah after the disappointment of 1999 and his cruel non-selection in 2003. We were so driven to be in the best shape possible that it must have made for some interesting sights. Whether in the gym or interval training around Logan Park, we were like Apollo Creed and Rocky on the beach, refusing to give any yards to each other. It was beneficial. We had fitness testing in Christchurch at the first All Blacks camp. I was pretty quiet for the first few days, ready to face the consequences but not wanting to put my head above the parapet after my unsanctioned trip to Fiordland. Thankfully, I finished with test results that were better than my best the year before. I'm unashamed to admit that I felt pretty chuffed about that, and felt that perhaps the sword hanging over my head had been removed. But word had got around that I'd missed the first week of the conditioning window and I believe a few of the boys were pretty pissed off with me. Ted made a point of pulling me aside and reminding me how much everybody had at stake.

I came back to Super Rugby against the Cheetahs in Invercargill. Normally you come back after a layoff and you're rusty and struggling to suck in deep breaths, but I remember in that game feeling so good. The conditioning must have worked, because the game felt like a canter and even if the Cheetahs weren't one of the stronger South African sides, at the very least you normally felt like you'd been in a physical battle.

This feeling extended through to the Tri Nations. We were so fit and sharp it almost felt like we were unbeatable. When we played and beat the Boks in Durban they were commenting after the game that it felt like we had half a step on them all across the field.

By that stage, I don't think anybody was under any illusion as to what the World Cup meant to the coaching staff. If anything, the whole thing had become a bit claustrophobic. The leadership group, which had started off with great intentions, had now become a bit of a grind. I hasten to say that I'm talking from my own perspective here, but to me it felt like the concept had already lost its way and needed refining.

When it started, we were laser-focused and totally process driven, which was driven by Wayne Smith and Bert Enoka. There was tension and nervous energy about the World Cup, but as a group we knew what we had to do and knew we had the tools to do it.

We had four pillars: preparation; focus on the now, not the past or the future; exert physical dominance through technique and strength; express yourself by being yourself. This last point sounds like cereal-box psychology, but it was actually a bit of a departure from the norm. As All Blacks, your personality is often suppressed by this idea that you had to act a certain way — that you're this strong, silent type who followed orders and ate, slept and drank rugby. We wanted to dismantle that, to an extent. This is going to sound really stupid, but it could be as simple as waving to people from the team bus. When I first made the All Blacks and became aware of people watching us as we left or arrived at the ground, I honestly didn't wave back to people because I wondered if it wasn't the done thing. I thought we had to be so single-minded and focused on the game that it would be seen by the older guys as a sign you weren't properly switched on. We decided we wanted to wave to people if we felt like engaging, not act so super serious because that's what was expected. We felt that the confidence you had in feeling able to express your personality would flow on to decision-making on the field. We didn't want robots: we wanted rugby players.

Somewhere along the way, however, we started over-complicating it for ourselves. The leadership group became a beast we kept having to feed, even when it wasn't hungry. We lost focus.

You know the old joke about government department bureaucrats holding meetings to arrange meetings? It started to feel a bit like that. We were flying around the country to talk about exactly the same things we had talked about in the previous meeting, and we'd finish off by arranging to meet again.

Handing a portion of the responsibility for the team back to the players was a great idea. It was forward thinking by Ted, Shandy and the management team. But with new approaches come new wrinkles, and I think they started to show themselves at the worst possible time. The off-field behaviour had improved, there was certainly a lot more scrutiny among the players as to what was the right mix of socialising and the hard work, but in terms of helping to set strategic and tactical direction, I felt the leadership group really just acted as rubber-stampers of Ted's theories rather than actually testing and challenging him. There weren't rifts, but things were fraying. It was fast becoming a chore rather than an honour.

Which is where we come, finally, to Game Plan Two.

We'd only experienced three defeats in the previous three seasons, but one of them was a 15–20 loss to the Wallabies in Melbourne in World Cup year and it spooked Ted. We had a leadership group meeting just prior to the World Cup, and the coaches expressed concern that the rest of the world was catching up to our plan of playing with pace and width. They decided we needed Game Plan Two (GPT).

GPT was going to hinge around forward-dominated, mauling, pick-and-go rugby. It would be exactly what I ended up playing at Toulon. It would only be used for the knockouts, when the rugby tightened up and became more about avoiding mistakes. During pool play, we were continuing to play with speed, to beat teams with footwork, and employ an intensity other teams couldn't live with. We had a strong set piece and tactical nous at first-five from DC and Nick Evans, who was such an underrated No. 10 — perhaps a player who in any other generation would have played a lot more games. We could run from everywhere, but we had a strong kicking game, too.

We breezed through Italy in Marseille and put 100 points on Portugal in Lyon. That game saw me come off the bench and play lock, as we were a bit short in the second row. After the game, the Portuguese took on our dirt trackers in football and gave us a right towelling, putting at least 10 goals on us, so a bit of balance was restored.

We crossed the Channel to play Scotland, who chose to run a virtual 2nd XV against us, which was disappointing, and then were too good for Romania in Toulouse. We won our pool convincingly, which set up a bizarre quarter-final with the hosts, France, who had lost their opener to Argentina to finish second in their pool. Unbelievably, the game would be played in Cardiff because, to guarantee their votes to host the Cup, the French organising committee had promised matches to Wales and Scotland. There was already chatter in the media that the French were going to suffer the indignity of being knocked out of their 'home' World Cup on foreign soil, which was presumptuous in the extreme.

With pool play done and dusted, we prepared to radically change our game plan, a move designed to catch our opposition by surprise. All it really achieved was to muddy our own waters. We were going to play a French team in a mauling game that is the bread and butter of their Top 14 club competition.

A fully functioning, mature leadership group, the sort that emerged in the years to follow, would have put the kibosh on it, but if I remember correctly, only Aaron Mauger expressed any real concern, and I'm not sure he did that with the coaches present. I know I didn't think it was a smart move, but I didn't want to rock the boat. If I had my time again, I would have said what I felt, namely that we should have the alternative game plan up our sleeves and change for short periods during a game, but then come back to the width and space game. It seemed extraordinary to me that we'd been so successful for three and a half years, yet we were pinning our World Cup on an unproven plan.

The odd feeling, the sense that all wasn't right, bled into other aspects of the week. During pool play, we didn't do a lot of contact training, but leading into the Cardiff quarter-final, guys like Xavier Rush, who was playing in Wales, came in with some others and we had a full 15-on-15 contact training.

This is totally my reading of it, but even Smithy seemed befuddled by what was going on. He was always so precise and pinpoint, but his expertise was nullified by these tactics. His video presentations were always excellent and engaging, using contemporary footage to perfectly illustrate the point he was making. That week, he was using footage from years previous and the points he was making seemed less razor sharp than normal. It seemed so un-Smithy-like.

Again, this isn't all on the coaches. If the leadership group was working the way it should have been, we would have aired our concerns and been more forthright. But because we'd been so successful, nobody wanted to be the one who questioned the direction we were heading. The concept had worn so thin by then and I don't think it's any coincidence that a lot of the guys in the group were gone at the end of the World Cup.

There was also an arrogance in the selection. I mean no offence to the people who were selected, because they were all there on merit, but Keith Robinson hadn't played a full game of rugby for a long time yet here he was being picked to start at the sharp end of the world's biggest tournament. Unless you're Jonah, you can't do it, especially if you're a forward.

After Tana's departure, we still hadn't picked our man at centre. Conrad Smith was there, but he was fairly inexperienced, so when it came to the quarter-final we picked Mils Muliaina at No. 13. I've since heard that Wayne Bennett, the legendary league coach, was involved in the tournament debrief and one of the most pointed questions he asked was why you'd pick one of the best fullbacks in the world at centre. It was a question he could have asked in 1999 and 2003 as well.

World Cup-winning sides are stable. Aaron Mauger was in the stands, as was Chris Jack. Chris had been a big part of the team for a long time, and he was completely forgotten about. They wanted Keith's physical edge against a team like France that could push the boundaries, but it's hard to provide that when you haven't been on the field.

I can only remember patches of the game and even those patches aren't in sharp focus. It was heartbreaking. Three years of work and you could sense it slipping away.

People got stuck into Anton for his war analogy — he said that the post-match dressing room had the stench of death, like a World War I battlefield — and although the imagery sounded over the top, I knew exactly what he meant. To call it a hollow feeling wasn't enough. I've never been in a dressing room like it before or since.

I didn't know what to do, so I called my dad. He was on a flight from New Zealand that had just landed. He was there, like hundreds of other New Zealanders, for the semi-finals and final.

'Dad,' I said. 'I've got some bad news. We lost tonight.'

'You get another go, don't you?' he replied.

He knew how the tournament worked, but right at that moment he couldn't comprehend it.

My mum and sisters were holidaying around France. We were all meeting in Paris that week. All our plans, shattered.

Everyone in the team just wanted to dig a hole and disappear. I felt sorry for Richie having to face the media while we just slunk around in our own misery.

Talk started to bubble away about the ref, Wayne Barnes, but I didn't hold anything against him. I did question how he got the game, because it was obvious he was very fresh and couldn't make a decision, but it didn't alter the fact we were poor.

We couldn't get out of the country until the following Thursday. It was a nightmare for Shandy, dealing with 36 angry and devastated footy players who had their eyes set on doing well for their country but who ended up feeling they were the worst team ever. Doug Howlett hit the headlines for jumping on cars at Heathrow while he was pissed, but there were a lot of guys letting off steam in unhealthy ways.

I ended up flying back into Christchurch and the next day my grandfather passed away. Dropped dead on the farm. I said to Nana that he must have been pissed off with our performance. I was in an emotional fog and his death quickly put things in perspective. He was the rock of the family in many ways. Mum and my sisters had to cut their holiday short to come home. The end of that trip was vastly different to what they'd bargained for.

Meanwhile, Sky was showing endless reruns of the game. I avoided them. I didn't need to see Game Plan Two ever again.

9

ŌPUNAKE, 2022, MY FALSE FRIEND

IN OCTOBER LAST YEAR, 2022, a cop car pulled in behind me as I turned into the driveway of the family farm at 4745 South Road. I was asked to do an evidential breath test. There was no suspense for me as I blew into the machine and waited for the reading to come back. I knew it wasn't a matter of whether I was over the limit, but by how much. Quite a bit, as it turns out — 1016 micrograms of alcohol per litre of breath, more than four times the legal driving limit. The cop, a local Ōpunake constable, was pretty understanding. He could see I wasn't in good shape and was asking me if I was on my medication. It was cordial enough. I wasn't trying to duck and dive or make a run for the house.

In the swirl of emotions that takes hold when you've been caught doing something stupid, it's not always the right one you land on first. I should have felt ashamed, or at the very least contrite, but the first thing I felt was self-pity: how unlucky was I to have been picked up drink-driving in coastal Taranaki, where cops are scarce and mostly unobtrusive? The second thing I felt was anger, because I learned luck had nothing to do with it. It was my partner Kiko who had called the police on me. What kind of betrayal was that?

That's the thing with the booze, though. It warps your perception of reality. It heightens your sensitivities and deregulates your emotional response to things. When the fog cleared, I realised that Kiko hadn't acted out of spite, but to protect the community and me. It's one thing to get in a car drunk and endanger yourself. It's another to put other people at risk.

I was duly charged with driving under the influence (DUI) and some of those close to me were encouraging me to seek name suppression. Legal advice suggested that because of my mental instability, there was a good chance I could make a successful application to keep my name out of the public domain. In the end I just thought: 'Fuck it. I did it, I made a choice to do it, I have to face up to the penalty.' I don't mean that to sound noble, because there is nothing noble about getting behind the wheel pissed, but I just didn't want to worm my name out of a bad situation. It wasn't nice seeing my name in the papers again, with all the same missteps in my life rehashed. I was momentarily pissed off because there had been no reporters at court, so someone must have fed them the story afterwards. But there again I'm getting angry at the wrong people, rather than looking at the root cause of the distress: me and my relationship with alcohol. The DUI, the misplaced anger, the court case: that was a dark couple of days. Another setback on this bumpy journey of mine.

There were a lot of things leading to this point — Mum's death earlier in the year, my inability to work for any period of time without the sense that I was frying my brain and my increasingly uncertain future — but the decision to drink on that day was mine, as was the decision to get behind the wheel of a car. Rather than look to apportion blame or to duck the embarrassment of having my name in the news for all the wrong reasons, I had to own that. More importantly, I have to own this simple, four-word sentence.

I am an alcoholic.

There, I've said it. When I read back on this, or my kids read it, or my friends that see only my best side, that sentence is going to hit like a thud, but it's true. I've been part of 12-step programmes, counselling and rehabilitation. I've been to meetings in France and in New Plymouth. It's an ongoing process. When I drink, I don't regulate my intake and in turn

I can't regulate my emotional response. If you combine it with my neurodegenerative disease, it's a toxic cocktail, if you'll excuse the pun.

I might not be the sort of alcoholic who wakes up in the morning and craves it. I can and have gone for long periods without any desire to drink, but the disease nevertheless presents as a day-by-day battle to stay out of its grip. It once would have given me great embarrassment to acknowledge any alcohol problems, but now I've come not only to accept it but also to understand that talking about it helps. I do get pissed off and I'll push back when people imply that my dementia and probable CTE is the result of alcohol, because I know a whole lot of players in similar positions to me who were at worst moderate drinkers during their careers. Still, I know it's a cog in my wheel. I drank most weekends, like a lot of teammates and fellow professional rugby players in that era, when the game became awash with money but the amateur ethos still held firm in many respects. It has become an all-too-convenient scapegoat for rugby officials to point the finger at alcohol when all evidence points to repetitive head impacts as the single most important and plausible cause of CTE. That aside, it has had negative health and social outcomes for me in myriad ways.

I've been, in one way or another, surrounded by a culture of drinking my entire life. It was nobody's choice but mine, but I fitted right into it, embraced it, even. My alcohol history is also a potted history of my life. I don't blame anybody else except me for taking things to extremes, but one of the reasons I want to tell my story is because alcoholism can be an insidious disease. It certainly was in my case. It was a thirst slaker, a social lubricant, a rite of passage, a male-bonding facilitator, a provider of Dutch courage, a relaxant, a stress reliever, a pain reliever, a sleep assister. Before I knew it, alcohol had become the answer to everything — and it was never the right answer.

In the weeks after that DUI idiocy, I slipped off the wagon again. I had a full-blown mental breakdown that I will talk about later, which was either exacerbated by alcohol or led me to drink again. It doesn't really matter which way around it happened: it's the inextricable link between alcohol and my mental health that is the critical point. It caused me to fly into a rage. I didn't hurt anybody except myself and some walls, but this is where I'm at. It's not pretty, it's not sustainable and I wish to god it was easy to stop harming myself in this way. In the cold light of day, it is so simple to sit back and say: 'Right. You've learned your lesson (again). This is it. No more drink.' But as soon as something triggers my emotions in a negative way, drinking is the first thing I think about doing. It's a vicious cycle that always ends up at the same start and end point: anger and self-loathing.

I hope when you're reading this book I haven't had a drink in months, but I can't promise you that. I know that alcohol doesn't do me any favours. After I've been drinking, I still have all the symptoms of my dementia, but it's like they're on steroids. I get depressed, my anxiety goes through the roof and my cognitive function is even worse than normal.

The longest stint I've been without a drink since my first foray during my 1st XV years was about a year. That was in my Ironman days when I was super fit and a lot of my spare time was taken up either in the pool, the ocean, on a bike or running the roads. I can't tell you if I missed it or not, or if my life was markedly better or not, because the key for me really was that I just wasn't thinking about it. Although it sounds pessimistic — defeatist, even — being off the drink doesn't dramatically improve my life. There's no great clarity or reawakening. Life is just 'less worse'. Last summer, for example, when I was close to a year sober, I'd come off the boat after skippering a couple of charter cruises and was in a really bad place. Kiko was worried about me because she said I'd just get home and get this vacant look. Life was going on around me, but I wasn't contributing. I'd just stare out the window. My kids would be talking to me but I was incapable of responding. They'd say: 'Daddy's gone off to Daddyland.' It's heartbreaking, really: you desperately want to be a vital part of these people's lives, but you're in a place where no one can reach you and you have no idea how to snap out of it.

Mum died in March 2022, and alcohol started sneaking back into my life. Hers was a horrible, slow death from a brain tumour, and I was a close witness to her last weeks and months.

It affected me deeply, but it feels selfish to say that: she was the one going through the pain and the realisation she wouldn't have a long life as a doting grandmother. I should have been grieving, but my stunted emotional range wouldn't allow it. I was probably feeling: Who gives a shit how I feel about it?

Drinking became a familiar and comforting emotional crutch. Not full-blown, bottle-of-spirits-a-night shit, like I got myself into in those dark, dark days in Pau, but I'd finish a day working on the boat and think it would be a good idea to prise open a couple of beers or bottles of wine. Kiko didn't think I could manage that, and she's right, so I started attending meetings again to keep on an even keel — a boat reference that seems pretty appropriate, given the circumstances.

So I'm waging a daily battle and have reached a position where I know things can go from being okay to going badly really, really quickly. I'm doing the best I can. It's something I need to continue working on daily: to get rid of that sense of uselessness and worthlessness that leads me to think it can be solved temporarily by ripping the top off a few beers.

That's where I am now. I'm older but not necessarily wiser, and when I look back at my life and my choices around alcohol, I can see how the environments you're in can shape your attitudes. Again, the choices I've made are all mine, but this is how I got there.

* * *

Growing up in a rural environment, I watched Mum and Dad work bloody hard. Much of my work ethic I put down to their influence. It was a really tight-knit farming community full of family and friends around Oaonui and Ōpunake.

Most weekends there seemed to be a party or a function of some sort that we would be dragged willingly along to. All the kids would play together as the adults had their fun. Although we were close-knit, we were still flung pretty wide and there were no taxis and Uber wasn't even a twinkle in some American billionaire's eye. The rule of thumb was whoever could walk the straightest would drive home. Us kids would be in the back seat and our job was to look out for the police. Dad would tell us to let him know straight away if we saw them. As a kid, there was a bit of humour to it all, but of course, you don't understand the potential seriousness of someone having a crash.

There'd be a bit of chat when somebody from around the region ended up in a ditch but it was only really when my sister Becky ended up in a wheelchair that it all came home to us how fragile life is. She wasn't driving — there was a sober driver — but she was drunk in the passenger seat and had her feet up on the dash when the driver fell asleep and crashed.

One of the phrases I heard often when I was a kid was that so-and-so needed 'a good blowout'. That was how you resolved stuff when you were too uptight, stressed or overworked. You had a blowout on the booze. That binge drinking was normalised and even seen as a healthy way of letting off steam, a reward for hard work. The farmers worked extremely hard; they let off steam hard, too.

Dad was big into home brewing. Down the coast, we had these things called 'discussion groups'. The farmers would take turns inviting others around to their place, give them a tour of the property and talk about the various techniques or innovations they were using to try to boost production. It would always be accompanied by a crate or two or three of beer. Dad proudly unleashed his home brew on the discussion group, and it was obviously a bit more potent than the usual staples like DB Draught, Double Brown or Lion Red, because there were about five or six farmers who were subsequently banned by Mum from ever darkening Dave Hayman's doorway again. To be fair, I'm not sure there were many queuing up to try Dad's brew again, anyway.

My drinking career didn't start until I got to Dunedin and made the 1st XV at King's. It was all pretty light-hearted stuff and I imagine pretty standard around school rugby at the time. The boys would play a game and occasionally one of the country boys in the team would invite everyone out for a few drinks and a bit of a knees-up in the woolshed. There'd be a keg involved and it'd be a pretty sociable time. When I hosted, Mum would always put a big pot of mince on the stove and serve it with white bread and spuds to make sure everyone had food in their stomachs. It was a way of bonding with your teammates, to get to understand the various walks of life that make up a team. Yeah, sure, you might have a few chuckles at school the next week if someone had one too many, but I can't honestly look back at these sessions with anything but fondness. Nearly everyone in the team was involved and they didn't end up like me, so it wasn't like these 1st XV excursions were a gateway to alcohol abuse. But drinking certainly did seem like a way to bring people together, and that notion persisted into my club and NPC days.

I left school and joined Southern, and I've already mentioned coach Steve Hotton's mantra, which was the classic 'play hard, drink hard' mentality. I played my first game for Southern and then underwent my initiation at the Fitzroy Hotel. I had to do a jug skol, which was standard enough fare, but one of the more senior members of the team said another tradition was having to snort a shot of chartreuse up my nose. If you're not familiar with green chartreuse, it's a particularly potent French herbal liqueur that comes in at an eye-popping 55 per cent alcohol by volume. Nose-shredding might be a better way to describe it. It was the most horrible drinking experience of my life.

I could do a nifty jug skol back in my day. In that manly, testosterone-fuelled environment, you got kudos for it. I don't mind admitting I'd feel a bit of pride when I'd overhear people say: 'Man, did you see Zarg do that jug?' It became part of who I was. I was the young guy who proved himself by being able to drink like a fish and turn up to training the next day and out-train everybody. I had this thing where I liked proving to teammates that I could push through and could shake off whatever dust I'd collected the night before. The scary thing for me is I often wonder what my potential would have been if I'd lived a more restrained life.

At this stage of my life, I wasn't drinking every weekend, but I was laying the foundation. The approval I was getting convinced me this was a path worth pursuing. And it wasn't difficult. Otago had a Speight's liaison officer who travelled with the team. His job was to make sure that every town we went to we could find either a Speight's bar or a bar serving it, so we kept the team's major sponsor happy. The brainwashing worked on us. Speight's was a Lion Breweries product, so anything made by Dominion Breweries became known as the Devil's Urine. The lines could become a little blurred when you travelled to Australia, for instance, where Lion had the licence for Heineken, but DB had it in New Zealand. The consequences were dire if you were caught drinking Devil's Urine, because the only way to rid it from your body was via a purge. That basically involved skolling as many jugs as it took for you to chunder. If the vomit was not deemed to be of acceptable volume, you would have to keep going. Only then could you claim to have been exorcised and admitted to a church (a Speight's pub) again. When I tell Kiko this story, she thinks it's horrific, and while she's right, I have to confess

I quite enjoyed the structure these rules and rituals gave to our social life.

For home games, you'd shower up and there were always a few beers in the sheds. Then we'd hit the supporters' club and do the rounds there, drinking and listening to the speeches. Then the call would be made to go back to the changing sheds, where we'd wheel out a keg and enjoy a court session. You didn't have to have played badly or done anything notably foolish to cop a fine. Any player who was on the cover of the programme would have to do a jug. It was a lot of fun, and if you split a keg between 30-odd players and 10 coaching and management staff, it was basically a jug each. We'd drain the keg and head into town, before turning up for a well-named recovery session the following morning.

It was a curious time in rugby's history. We were getting paid to play but we still carried over many of the amateur traditions. There was this transition period and I was smack bang in the middle of it at Otago. I embraced that Southern Man ethos as espoused in the Speight's ads. I was the real-life embodiment of it with my farming background, big frame and scruffy beard. My behaviour fitted that cliché, too. I remember a commentator once describing me as 'looking like I'd just emerged from the Catlins, where I'd been feeding on possum'. I didn't run from that. I never sought out the spotlight, but there was part of me that probably enjoyed that whiff of notoriety. It wasn't an affectation, but it also wasn't all there was to me.

I did nothing to dissuade people from the belief, however, that I spent my non-rugby waking hours in a Swanndri and Red Bands, shooting wild pigs and drinking Speight's.

At the Highlanders, coach Peter Sloane thought it'd be a great idea to bring a breathalyser to the recovery session following games. He did it with the best of intentions, to try to get us to ease back on the post-match celebrations, to demonstrate how a big night was still affecting your sobriety the following day. Instead, we soon corrupted it for our own ends. It quickly became a challenge to see who could blow over 1000 micrograms. That was when the machine gave up. You'd get all these players lining up and if the player blew 1000 there'd be cheers and if you finished short the place would ring out in boos. I don't think it pleased the management that much, but that was our attitude to anybody trying to inhibit our post-match revelry.

I should note that it wasn't like this *every* weekend. There were sometimes periods of up to a month where I'd stay off the booze because we had a run of big games coming up. But the connection between rugby and drinking was pretty pervasive. I know I'm not alone in paying the price now. There's a few guys from that era who have struggled with alcohol during and post their careers and have found themselves in trouble in one way or another. Again, we're all responsible for our actions, but there are some interesting cultural factors as to why it was perhaps easier than it should have been to get into that state where your relationship with alcohol is unhealthy and even dangerous.

Otago was a bit different, too. Eroni Clarke came down to the Highlanders for a season in 2002 and I remember him telling me he couldn't believe what he was seeing. He'd played with guys who were no shrinking wallflowers on the drink at Auckland and the Blues, but he reckoned that what he encountered in Dunedin was next-level. You'd think it would be a bit embarrassing to hear that, especially coming from somebody who had been a big part of winning teams in Auckland and knew how a high-performance environment should work, but no. It mostly felt like a badge of honour.

Part of that was the social environment we were in. Many of us were students — I was studying at Otago Polytech — and we were living in New Zealand's ultimate university town. You had the classic scarfie pubs like the Cook, the Gardies and the Bowler — all gone now — and if you think the rugby players were bad... We mainly limited our socialising to a Saturday night, but those places were heaving from Wednesday night onwards through the weekend. If CTE really is associated with alcohol, then there should be a bunch of Otago students from the '90s wandering around with severe neurological problems! As young footy players with a bit of cash at hand, we were swept up in that maelstrom and it was a rewarding time. The beers no doubt provided a bit of Dutch courage, too, if you were trying to impress the female students. As a shy country kid who was never going to be mistaken for Brad Pitt, I needed all the help I could get in that department.

When I got a bit of money coming in, I bought a house in St Clair, a beachside suburb in Dunedin's south, across the road from the surf club on Victoria Road. In 2002, the same year Clarke came down for his eye-opening season at the Highlanders, I had my King's and Southern mate Warren Moffat, former Counties first-five Blair Feeney, and North Harbour halfback Billy Fulton living with me. We decided we were going to get into home brewing and got pretty serious about it. Even in summer — or what passes for a summer in Dunedin — we had the fires going in the lounge to keep the room temperature at optimum level. We made more quart bottles of the stuff than we could count. Anton Oliver was recovering from an injury — it might have been his Achilles — and dropped around to my place for a brew. He was obviously impressed and told the rest of the boys that he felt it had some medicinal properties and that was all we needed for the place to turn into what was known as the Victoria Tavern.

We ended up proudly taking crates of the stuff in for a team court session and joked that we wanted to move in on Speight's territory. If memory serves me, everybody was meant to do a jug skol, but the crates had been shaken up in transit and it was a fairly cloudy, uninviting soup that we were forcing people to drink. Not the best advert for our hard work, perhaps, but with hazy ales being all the rage these days, I suppose you could say we were craft brewers ahead of our time.

Mad Monday or end-of-season sessions were always eagerly anticipated. Tony Brown had a Nifty Fifty scooter that would be wheeled out for the occasion, so there would invariably be time trials, often involving nudity, around a greasy Carisbrook track. The Otago Rugby Union was based at the ground in those days, so all the office staff there would have seen things they probably would have preferred not to.

It was only once Ted Henry came in at the All Blacks in 2004 that I really experienced any moderation of the drinking culture. There was a consensus that our attitudes to alcohol and to recovery had to change. Guys heading out in cliques looking for a good night had been replaced by more organised team events by the social committee. Ali Williams was known as a fine lock outside the team, but inside the squad he was better known as the guy who could unlock the doors to pubs and clubs in Auckland where we could relax as a team. Partners and wives started to become more involved, which might have been anathema to previous generations, but was actually a really positive development. Young men aren't great at talking amongst themselves about things beyond the footy field, but in this more inclusive, family environment, you actually got to know your teammates and the things that were important to them.

We weren't perfect. It wasn't like we ended every night out holding hands and singing 'Amazing Grace'; there were still big,

big nights and sorry mornings. Still, we were making a dent in that all-consuming, 'play hard, drink hard' ethos. I talked to Andrew Hore about this once when I had left for Europe and he had stayed on in New Zealand for another World Cup cycle. When we were cutting our teeth in footy, those who didn't drink or even those who did have a couple of beers but never got drunk were in the absolute minority. If you were on tour anywhere, domestically or overseas, and wanted to find a teammate or two to go and grab a beer with, it was never difficult. He was telling me that by the time he finished his career, it was almost the opposite. The young players coming through hadn't been exposed to that clubrooms' drinking culture that used to govern the game.

That's a good thing, I think, but it was too late for me.

* * *

When I got to Newcastle, I noticed an immediate change in the drinking culture. Now don't get me wrong: Newcastle is a party town. It's famous for women's skirts getting shorter the colder it gets, and Osborne Road in the Jesmond district is stag and hen party heaven. Natalie went out for a girls' night there shortly after we arrived, and got togged up in her best party clothes. She came back in the early hours exclaiming that she was overdressed and could not believe how much and how fast the girls drank.

Within the team it was different. We had Jonny Wilkinson and Toby Flood, who didn't drink at all, and there were no court sessions or any real team bonding over alcohol as such. You'd play your game, you might have a couple of drinks afterwards and then everybody would tend to drift off either in small groups or on their own to catch up with friends outside of rugby.

As a result, we kind of had a clique of Kiwi boys. Guys like myself, Brent Wilson, Tane Tu'ipulotu and Joe McDonnell would hang out and drink together. We even had the great idea of ordering a pallet of Speight's from the people who ordered the beer for all the Walkabout pubs in London. In case you're wondering, no, we didn't drink it all ourselves. If we were playing, say, Leicester, we'd get in touch with Aaron Mauger and have a couple of slabs put aside for him. We did it all at cost, so we weren't a black market Speight's operator, but the whole thing worked out to be about 70p a stubbie — much cheaper than drinking at a pub! Guinness sponsored the premiership in those days and there were always a couple of dozen in the changing rooms. The black stuff is fairly divisive amongst high-performance athletes, so much of it would go untouched and always seemed to find its way into the back of McDonnell's car, which was handy.

In Toulon, again, there was no culture of team drinking or court sessions. Alcohol was a part of French life but their attitude was that it was an adornment to the evening, not the reason for it. It took me a while to get my head around the concept of aperitifs — a drink before food, the most traditional being the anise-flavoured pastis — and digestifs like cognac that were 'taken' after dinner. But as you can imagine, I enjoyed learning.

There was such a high turnover among the players in my first few years there that it was hard to get any sort of team spirit, but barbecuing started to play an important role. We'd gather on a Sunday for a barbecue and beers and the French guys would start talking to the English-speaking guys and gradually we actually got to know our teammates as more than players with a number on their back. We also started picking up more and more of each other's language, by osmosis more than anything. I don't want to give alcohol too much credit, but the atmosphere at the club definitely improved. Chris Masoe, the All Black flanker, had a great place with a pool and we'd frequently entertain our French-speaking teammates there on a Sunday afternoon.

Unfortunately, it was at Toulon where my drinking started to become problematic. Well, I'll rephrase that: it was already problematic, but it was there where it started to have ramifications beyond my own personal health. Those Saturday-night sessions after a game had started to bleed into the Sunday barbecues, but I still prided myself on going into the club on Monday morning and working harder and better than anybody else. What I was slow to pick up on was the damage it was doing to my marriage. I was stupidly selfish and stubborn about it. I had the whole: 'Hey, you knew who I was before you married me, so if you suddenly don't like it, too bad' crap going on. I'd keep coming up with bullshit justifications why I needed to be with the boys drinking — I was 'a team leader', 'I was improving the club culture' — but really, it was just placing my personal enjoyment above the wants and needs of my family.

Jesus, I cringe when I think about it now, but that's how my mind worked. You know, I functioned like that my whole career. Train the house down, play my guts out on a Saturday then hit the piss as a self-serving reward. I couldn't count how many Saturday nights I've returned home with varying levels of drunkenness, from remembering getting in a taxi to waking up and seeing my car in the driveway and having to do a circuit of it to check for dents and paint scrapings, all the while hoping it was someone sober who had driven me home while fearing it could have been me behind the wheel.

Am I proud of that? If it sounds like I am, then rest assured I'm not. It's shit behaviour, but again, it's best if I don't sugar-coat it. There's no point in me giving you a sanitised version of myself.

There's also a question of why nobody stepped in before I started hurting myself, but the answer is twofold: throughout my career, I tended to gravitate towards people like myself, drinking buddies or people who, for some reason, liked my company on the drink; and people, especially Nat, were in their own ways trying to make it clear that my drinking was not normal, but I wasn't ready to listen.

Towards the end of my career at Toulon, ironically the 'glory years' of my career, I was also dealing with something else: constant pain. It's not an excuse, but I was justifying a lot of my drinking as self-medication. My back, with bulging discs, was giving me a lot of grief, and I played the last seasons of my career with no skin on the end of my nose, an injury that would need a graft when I finished. Getting in the shower was so painful, but there was a paradox at play here, because I also took great pleasure in the pain. I enjoyed waking up on a Sunday morning feeling like I'd been 12 rounds with Mike Tyson, because I told myself that meant I'd done my job. If others weren't feeling the same way as me, it was because they hadn't gone as hard as me. If it meant I just had to have a few extra beers or another bottle or two of wine that day to dull the pain, then that was a price I was willing to pay.

The pain was my friend initially. My scars and herniated discs were my calling cards. After a while, it became something else, however. It started to mess with me psychologically. Up until then, I'd largely been a weekend drinker. In my later years at Toulon, I'd started to drink midweek. More worryingly, I guess, I started drinking on my own. Nat would go to bed and I'd sit up for a couple of hours with just wine for company. Whereas I'd been able to justify the way I drank before as nothing abnormal in my circles, I now started to realise that staying up on my own to drink enough to get to sleep without pain was abnormal, even by rugby standards. I also noticed my tolerance for alcohol was waning. I used to take a weird sort of pride in the amount I could drink before it had a noticeable effect on me. Now I was getting drunk more quickly and failing to recognise it, let alone the damage it was doing around me.

My marriage was breaking down. When I look back, it shouldn't have been a surprise. Nat was travelling to New York for a holiday with her sister. I went to Nepal with Franck, so we had started expanding our interests in life and they didn't involve each other. There was a part of me that thought that everything would be fine once I retired. I wouldn't be dealing with the constant pain. I'd no longer have rugby as a justification for drinking, so I'd get on top of that side of my life, too. Instead, I found myself retired, with no money worries and not a lot to do, so I bought myself one of those perfect-pour beer machines. If the afternoon was nice, I'd sit myself in the garden and pour myself a couple of pints, maybe open a bottle of rosé, too.

Nat left me on my own for a week with the kids. I did everything I needed to do, but I was drinking to get myself through the night. I didn't have rugby as an excuse anymore, but I still used it as a justification. Hey, I played my heart out over more than 400 professional games. I have earned this life, and I deserve to take some time to relax. Me, me, me...

That's when things started to unravel. When I started to lose control.

As you know by now, I took a job in rugby when I swore I wouldn't and we moved to Pau.

It didn't go well then and, as I discover every time I make the decision to drink, it won't ever go well again if I choose alcohol.

This thing, this disease, is going to go one of two ways, and there's a lot to lose by going the wrong way.

10

NEWCASTLE, 2007–10, 'MILLION-DOLLAR' MAN

NAT AND I ARRIVED in Newcastle in the northeast of England for the last week of November 2007. My first impression was: 'Wow. It's 4 pm and it's dark.' It was dark and cold, really cold. I'd just come from the end of a New Zealand spring where, despite the World Cup result that had put the country in a collective bad mood, optimism was starting to rise along with the temperature. Being plunged back into the cold and dark sent our bodies into hibernation mode. We immediately had a craving for fatty foods. One night shortly after we'd arrived and settled in, we found ourselves sitting up in bed one evening eating from a bag of chips.

'What the hell are we doing?' Nat asked.

It was a valid question.

* * *

The year had been a weird one, what with the ill-fated World Cup campaign and the death of my grandfather. The latter had put the former into perspective. I knew that my career was short and that life was worth living.

After busting my gut for New Zealand Rugby over the past three years, I was in negotiations for a contract extension during 2007. I never expected to be offered the same as the numbers my agent, Warren Alcock, was receiving from clubs in Europe, but I did want recognition — without blowing my own horn, here — that I was one of the better tightheads in the world. I knew what kind of money the best tightheads were commanding in Europe and so did NZR, so no one was naïve from a financial point of view. I was a professional playing a professional game that was seeing increasingly large amounts of revenue. Although I would have taken less than what I could have to stay in New Zealand, I did want some acknowledgement of my value. That said, I was not a guy who found this sort of thing easy. I hated the idea of putting myself on a pedestal and I never sought out the sort of sponsorship deals and contra arrangements that others did because in my head, I thought who'd want a bushy-bearded bloke from Otago promoting their product (apart from Speight's, maybe)?

I reckon NZR knew this and played on it. They weren't dumb. They knew what the best tightheads, perhaps the most specialised, physically demanding position in rugby, were worth. It's a hard one for people to get their heads around, sometimes. Why does one of the most unglamorous positions on the park attract such a price premium? The best way I can explain it is that it is a technical position. If you're a loose forward or a midfielder, if you have athletic ability, you can essentially play it well from a really young age. There are nuances to those positions that you pick up through experience, but natural athleticism gets you a long way. A tighthead prop cannot be good on athleticism alone. It takes time to develop and mature. In that regard, you need people with the physical attributes to play the position — there are no light props like there are light centres, for example — and the really good ones have a mentality that drives them to impose themselves physically on every contest. It's not everyone's cup of tea.

There's nobody in the world who knows as much about scrums as Mike Cron, who has worked with World Cup-winning All Blacks and Black Ferns teams. He's got a great saying about the difference between a loosehead and a tighthead prop that I like to repeat whenever I get the chance (and with apologies to my great mate Tony Woodcock, who would beg to differ): 'A loosehead pisses with the wind at his back, a tighthead pisses into the wind.' That's because the axis of the scrum is on the hooker's right shoulder: my side of the scrum. 'If you haven't got a tighthead, you haven't got a scrum,' Cron would say.

Cronno is a great guy and a loyal friend. The tightheads he was used to seeing were great scrummagers, but some needed a wheelbarrow to get them from breakdown to breakdown. He took a liking to me because he knew I had a big engine around the park. He reckoned he'd never seen me completely physically spent, even after playing the full 80 in a Test match, which only proves that I must have been a decent actor. He also liked me, I suspect, because he saw me as a bit of a project. Tightheads were not meant to be tall like me, with long levers, so my set-up and technique had to be perfect. Initially, they were far from that. Another Cronno-ism is to talk about how it's easier to break a long broomstick across your knee than a short one. The problem with having a long femur, or thigh bone, like me, was that it was easier for my opposition to use it against me if I didn't have my angles absolutely spot on. We did a lot of work on set-up — 120-degree-angle knee-bend, feet a shoulder-width apart, equal weight going through each foot — until we got it close to perfect. 'A scrum is all about biomechanics,' Cron would say, describing it as like looking for the sweet spot when you're doing a squat lift, except you're doing it with your torso horizontal. At every scrum there's nearly three tonnes of pressure directed through your body, and it takes a certain breed to absorb that, put your head up and then run to the next breakdown. In short, a good tighthead is bloody hard to find. In Europe, where the scrum is king and so much strategic emphasis is placed on winning scrum penalties, the position is even more highly valued.

NZR knew this, but I was left feeling that they thought I'd take significantly less to play for the jersey. In other words, they treated me like I was dumb, and that didn't just leave a bad taste in my mouth, it pissed me off.

Word started to get out — leaked by them, I can only assume — that I had been offered a farm if I extended my contract and stayed. The number of questions I had to answer from journalists on that subject got on my nerves. It was a complete manipulation of the facts. It threw me under the bus and made me look grasping and selfish.

To put the record straight: New Zealand Rugby never offered to buy me a farm. I mean, that's just ridiculous. What Taranaki Rugby had offered was to pay the lease on a farm for me. That would have been the NPC component of my NZR contract, which was worth about $60,000 to $70,000 in those days. It was a tempting sweetener. I had made no secret that I felt my post-rugby future was on a dairy farm, but in no way was there ever the offer of buying me a farm, the value of which would have run into the millions.

I was even getting it from people I knew well. Shit like: 'Mate, they must be paying you a fortune up north if you can afford to turn down a farm.'

Perhaps I shouldn't have been so sensitive to it, but it got to the point where I wanted to get out of the country as fast as I could to leave all the talk behind. If you'd asked me then and there if I could see myself coming back, I'd have probably laughed in your face. But with a bit of distance and time, my mood towards New Zealand Rugby softened. But in the meantime, Nat and I packed our stuff up and headed away. It was an exciting time. She'd spent a long time living in Auckland and I was in Dunedin, so it had largely been a long-distance relationship.

The excitement barely outlived our arrival in Newcastle. It was a shock to the system. I'd already lived through Taranaki and Otago winters, so I thought I was fairly well insulated against the cold. But here I was training in thermals, a rugby jersey, a jacket and a beanie. Even on my coldest days in Dunedin, if you wore a jacket at training, you'd be seen as a bit soft. Here, in the frigid north of England, you had no choice.

But it wasn't just the weather. In New Zealand, I had come from a generic system of rugby. Whether it was the Highlanders, the All Blacks or even Otago, there was a system, especially with scrum techniques. Cronno's philosophies that were put in place at international level were passed down the chain — a case of trickle-down expertise. That meant there was continuity. I knew that when I played for the Highlanders, we were going to be doing the same thing at set piece, by and large, as we had in the ABs.

At Newcastle, suddenly, I was exposed. I was the new guy on the block expected to transform the fortunes of their pack, and yet I had to do it the way they wanted. It takes time to build respect for the people around you and for them to respect you. It doesn't matter what you're paid, you have to prove yourself, and that took a while.

The bedding-in process wasn't helped by a nagging feeling: for the first time in my life, I didn't feel like playing rugby. I'd put so much into the World Cup campaign and while I was keen to get out of New Zealand and the claustrophobic and angst-ridden reaction to the defeat, I'm not sure I was ready to lace the boots up again. I'd also spent a week with Andrew Hore on his farm tailing lambs, so I was pretty sore and knackered. A different environment was what I needed, but so was a decent break from footy.

Still, the money was nice, even if the obsession with it was a bit tiresome. Almost as soon as I signed with Newcastle, I started to see things appearing that I had become the highest-paid player in the world. I don't know if that was true and, even if it was, it wasn't really the ego boost you might think it should have been. For a start, the payment structure was actually a hell of a lot more complicated than simply signing a contract for X amount of pounds and getting a wodge of cash deposited into my account each week. If only it was that simple, or as sweet as it sounded in the British press when I arrived: 'Carl Hayman completed his far-fetched change of lifestyle yesterday, from chopping lambs' tails to becoming the most expensive player in British rugby on £6,500-a-week,' wrote veteran rugby writer Peter Jackson in the *Daily Mail*.

> Perhaps not surprisingly, given the therapeutic nature of his post-World Cup work on a farm 12,000 miles away, the bearded All Black giant sounded a touch sheepish about the size of a Newcastle contract understood to be worth some £75,000-a-year [more] than Jonny Wilkinson's at the same club…
>
> While Newcastle stress that the Northumberland countryside helped clinch the deal for the world's supreme tighthead prop by suiting his love of hunting, shooting and fishing, the sheer scale of the money on offer might just have had a bit to do with it.
>
> 'I guess I am surprised to some extent,' he said, referring to a deal which will earn him around £350,000-a-year for the next 30 months. 'Put it this way, I am not complaining. In world rugby, there's now more appreciation for the job front rowers do but I haven't really read much on the subject.

The club was actually in a bit of financial disarray when I arrived, and I can say hand on heart that the noises I received when I got there were along the lines of: 'We really didn't expect you to say yes to our offer.' They assumed that I'd either stay in New Zealand for the glory of playing for my country, or that I'd take the offer from Toulouse, who were an established powerhouse of European rugby.

Part of my contract was structured around image rights rather than salary. The club owned two image rights companies. I don't want to bore you with all the details of how it worked, but essentially they could put 33 per cent of your salary through each of their image rights companies, which meant they effectively paid half of my salary tax free. Every promotion you did for the club was documented, so it could be justified to Her Majesty's Revenue and Customs department.

Then the credit crunch hit and HMRC started clamping down on clubs. It was really messy. HMRC created new rules around image rights contracts, and they started going after players. I ended up paying tax on two-thirds of image rights and the only positive thing about that was that I hadn't already spent the cash on a house or a flash car. I was still doing all right, don't get me wrong, but the narrative around me being the highest-paid player in the world wasn't all it was cracked up to be by the media. There was no guarantee, also, that the taps wouldn't suddenly be turned off altogether. One of the club's biggest sponsors and benefactors, the Northern Rock bank, was nearly forced into insolvency as the global financial crisis hit. At one stage during my time there, we were brought into a meeting and told our salaries might not go in on the scheduled date because the club had no cashflow. That was pretty alarming, but luckily, the crisis was averted.

In my first full season, Newcastle was talking about offloading me to Johannsesburg-based Gauteng Lions for Currie Cup and Super Rugby so they could offset some of my salary. I was also looking at coming home. It was a real mess. We were struggling to get paid. It was unsettling, to the point where it seems a minor miracle that I saw out my three-year contract, let alone enjoyed it so much that I considered extending my stay there.

What I found was a club that had been stuck in its way of doing things for a long period of time. I don't know if they were resistant to change or had never really thought about it, but some of the things they were doing were substandard. The facilities weren't up to scratch. The gym had been kitted out in 1998 with a lot of techno-gym products and 10 years on, the machines were faulty or outright unusable. We had a gym full of stationary bikes with one pedal. I was coming from the New Zealand environment, where the teams had gyms with Olympic lifting platforms and weights; everything was in mint condition and well looked after by professionals. For somebody who loved the training aspect of rugby, to see how little investment Newcastle made compared to how much they invested in players like me was eye-opening and a little disappointing.

Our weight sessions were circuit training. For the forwards, a certain weight would be put on the bar and we'd run around the gym doing these circuits with set weights. I was pushing the same amount on each stand as an openside flanker, who clearly needed a different regime than I did. Nothing was tailored to the individual. There was very little monitoring going on and few players, if any, were keeping training diaries. I don't think there was any proper fitness testing. It was so foreign to me compared to what I had come from, but I didn't feel I could say anything because I knew how quickly I could turn from being Carl Hayman, the Test prop brought in to add starch to the pack, to Carl Hayman, the overpaid prima donna.

There was real instability in the coaching. When I arrived, John Fletcher was director of rugby and Peter Walton, an ex-Scotland international flanker, was the forwards coach. They didn't last long and Steve Bates, a former England scrumhalf, replaced Fletcher, but he too was gone at the end of the 2009–10 season. The captain was Phil Dowson, who played a few Tests for England and would also enjoy stints at Northampton and Worcester, which recently went bankrupt. In terms of leadership, the most ebullient figure at the club was a guy named Steve Black, who died in 2022 aged just 64. He was a local, a Geordie, and a famed motivator who had a particularly close relationship with our superstar flyhalf Jonny Wilkinson. Jonny and the rest of the boys loved Blackie, who always knew the right thing to say at the right time. His motivational skills were in hot demand, and he worked with Newcastle football legends like Alan Shearer as well.

On paper, we had a really good mix of players. We had a mostly English backline and until then, Newcastle had been notorious for playing a nice style of rugby, if lacking grunt up front. I was the hired grunt and it felt like a great opportunity to be a transformative type of player, although that brought with it some added pressure. Not that I was inclined to shy away from that: I'd played for the All Blacks for four straight years and had a pretty good handle on what pressure was.

On the loosehead side of the scrum was my old Otago sparring partner Joe McDonnell. He was one of the key spruikers to get me to Newcastle in the first place. While the Toulouse offer was attractive and the south of France might have had more sex appeal than the northeast of England, in the end, I didn't know the language or anybody there, so it was easier to imagine myself playing at Newcastle with an old mate propping up the scrum with me. We also had Mark Sorenson, a lock from Bay of Plenty. It took me a while to find my feet with the rest of my new teammates. I had a way of doing things, especially in the scrum, that didn't immediately gel with the rest. I needed to build respect.

My first game was away to Wasps, who had Lawrence Dallaglio, and Kiwis Riki Flutey and Joe Ward, and the remnants of the team that was European champion in 2007. They thumped us, which put our record at three wins and four losses. We then lost at home to Gloucester, so I had to wait until a couple of days before New Year's to get my first win for

Newcastle — away to Saracens — and my first win at all for what seemed a very long time.

In all reality, the primary goal that season was to avoid relegation, which we did comfortably enough because Leeds were so bad. But eleventh in the 12-team competition was not where Newcastle's owners expected to be, having invested so heavily in talent.

We stayed up north over the summer. I didn't want to return to New Zealand and go back-to-back-to-back winters. I bought a bright orange 1974 Volkswagen Kombi, put a board on the roof and drove it from Amsterdam across to France, down the Bay of Biscay to the Basque coast of Spain. We stayed at places like La Rochelle, Bordeaux and Biarritz. I loved the country and the coastline. No doubt it planted a seed in my mind about playing in France. At Biarritz, I caught up with Mike Clamp, the former All Black and Wellington wing, who ran a surf shop. They had a great little community there and I was a little jealous of the lifestyle.

The 2008–09 season started much as the last one had finished. We were competitive enough at our little Kingston Park home, but we tended to get our arses kicked on the road. By the time the year ended, I think we'd won two games, drawn one and lost six, so dreams of play-offs and qualifying for the Heineken Cup — the European championship — were put on hold as we went about the more sobering task of avoiding relegation.

It was then we started making significant changes at the club. To that point, we'd been travelling seven hours on a bus to Bath and would wonder why we didn't play with much zip. Get your atlas out and look where clubs like Gloucester, Bristol and Bath are located. Look at all the London clubs, like Wasps, Saracens, London Irish and Harlequins. Then trace your finger up the island to Newcastle to see the sort of distances we were travelling. Even the Midlands clubs, Northampton, Leicester and Worcester, were hours away.

We started flying and we started winning. In consecutive away games, we beat Bristol, Northampton and Sale, then got close to Bath and Wasps. We ended the season in tenth, still a really disappointing placing, but the nine wins and improved showing in the latter part of the season gave us confidence that we were on the cusp of turning Newcastle into a force.

* * *

At the World Cup, I had started playing guitar. It had occurred to me that I'd been going on all these rugby tours with a whole bunch of spare time, but I wasn't really doing anything with it. There were a couple of other guys who played, so I picked a guitar up one day and decided I was going to try to join the party. I got on YouTube and tried to teach myself.

When I got to Newcastle, I discovered Jonny Wilkinson was into his music, too. He was a good guitarist and pianist, so we'd head out to his place at Slaley Park, west of Newcastle, to jam. Jonny's brother Mark, known as Sparks, was a good drummer, and the team manager, John Stokoe, who was about our age, loved singing. We lacked a decent bass player. Toby Flood auditioned for a role a few times, but we didn't call him '12 Thumbs Flood' for no reason. We tried to nail all these British indie rock classics by the Arctic Monkeys and Milburn and a bunch of other bands I'd barely heard of before. It wasn't a weekly thing, but it was often enough that we started to develop some basic competencies and every now and then the call would go out for us to turn up in fancy dress. There's a picture somewhere of a six-foot-four Kiwi bloke with a bushy beard driving down the A69 in a bright orange Kombi dressed as a nun headed out to band practice.

This detour into the world of *Rolling Stone* magazine doesn't stop there. It turned out we weren't the only rugby crew in the UK who fancied their musical chops. There was a Māori fella called Brendon Daniel who left New Zealand really young to go to Saracens and played for a few clubs before ending up at Bath. He was a real talent, and ended up playing professionally on the Gold Coast — music, not rugby. Another guy, Spencer Davey, a centre, had come to Newcastle from Bath and was a friend of mine. He enjoyed a jam. We also had a lock, an ex-Royal Marine, called Andy 'Pez' Perry. Pez was a character with arms the size of tree trunks. He was so easy to wind up. You'd introduce him to people and say, 'Pez used to be in the army,' and he'd look you earnestly in the eye and say: 'It's not the army. It's the Royal Marines.' Needless to say, no one in the club was going to do anything but introduce him as having been in the army. Pez was a drummer.

The club found out about this hobby and asked us to play a concert for the supporters' club. It sounded like a great idea. We were to play in between our game and an England Six Nations Test later that evening. The club was packed, absolutely heaving, and it occurred to me I was far more anxious about getting up and playing a few songs in front of these people than I had been about playing the game I was well paid for earlier that day.

It went pretty well, but a secondary career as a rhythm guitarist was in no danger of taking off. Newcastle was probably the high point of my alternative rock aspirations: there's something about those cold and, at times, miserable places that draws you to music.

I need to quickly add that the miserable part of the equation relates directly to the weather. As a city, I really enjoyed the place and the people. It was a lot of fun. I lived in Jesmond Dene in an old stately home that had been chopped up into five apartments. Some of the apartments were used by people associated with the Newcastle football club. Tim Krul, the keeper, lived there but the highlight was when Paul Gascoigne moved in next door.

It was only for a short period of time, but he'd moved back to Newcastle to start working with their academy. He was a nice, chatty guy. I knew he had some demons, but he was always really pleasant around us, even if not entirely drama free. I was headed out to training one morning and the electric gates at the end of the driveway were swinging in the wind. I was wondering what was going on and then I saw Gazza around the side of the house and he's not in great shape. His face is a bit of a mess and he told me he'd been punched out by his old man. He'd lost a tooth and his house keys, which is why the gates were broken. Gazza was in a bit of a state, so I didn't know whether to leave him like that. In hindsight, I should have taken a bit more care of him, but I was running late for practice and by this stage Nat had come out to see what was happening.

He'd clearly had a big session and was saying: 'Oh, I've just had a bit of trouble with me dad.' Natalie took him in and made him a cup of tea and rang the Shepherds. Freddy Shepherd had been chairman of Newcastle for years, owned the properties and arranged for someone to come down, let Gazza into his apartment and help clean him up.

Later that night, there was a knock on the door and we answered it with a bit of trepidation. Gazza was standing there looking a bit sheepish. 'Hi Natalie. I just want to say thanks for looking after me. Thought it was the least I could do to give you some of these Indian takeaways.' We said thanks, waved him goodbye, opened the bag and yes, there was literally some half-eaten onion bhaji, samosas and a bit of naan. It all looked like it was a couple of days old, but thanks, Gazza!

That was a guy with a kind heart who was dealing with stuff a bit bigger than he was equipped to handle. I never got on the gas with Gazza, which was probably just as well, but I did see his mate Jimmy 'Five Bellies' Gardner come around and drop him off things in paper bags. Five Bellies had become almost as famous as Gazza himself, mainly for being the football star's fall guy. There were legendary stories, some with only a few small threads of truth: one about Jimmy letting Gazza burn his nose with a lighter for a £1000 bet; of Gazza tricking him into biting into a mince pie where he'd scraped out the filling and replaced it with cat excrement; of him swimming naked in the duck pond of a luxury London hotel; and yet another of Gazza buying an expensive robot and programming it to say: 'Make me a cup of tea, fat man.'

Gazza and Five Bellies were part of Newcastle folklore, and you could see why the people embraced them. People from Newcastle — Novocastrians — were always up for a drink, a laugh and never took themselves too seriously. Well, that's not quite true. When it came to football of the round-ball variety, they took themselves extremely seriously, that's for sure. I was fortunate enough to go along to St James' Park — what a cathedral that is — to watch the Magpies. It was hard not to get envious when you compared it to Kingston Park, which was our wee ground set out in a fairly unprepossessing, light industrial suburb on the outskirts of the city. St James' was an easy walk from the centre of the city and the atmosphere was never anything less than electric.

If the rugby club was in turmoil while I was there, it was nothing compared to the football club. Kevin Keegan, a beloved figure on Tyneside, had been appointed for his second stint as manager but resigned late in 2008 after a dispute with the club's board. His replacement, Joe Kinnear, then had a heart issue that forced him to stand down. That saw Alan Shearer, probably in a tie with Sting for the most famous Novocastrian of all time, take over on an interim basis. Newcastle were relegated on the last day of the 2008–09 season and there were literally grown men and women crying in the street, unable to process the fact they wouldn't be playing in the Premier League the next season. I guess it wasn't too different from some of those who flew to France to watch the All Blacks in the semi-finals and final of the 2007 World Cup, only to find out we'd been beaten in the quarters.

It wasn't just the people I loved about Newcastle. Northumberland is seriously underrated. It's a beautiful part of England and I used to spend quite a bit of time up the coast surfing. I can tell you that the North Sea is six degrees in winter and there wasn't a pair of board shorts in sight.

There were a bunch of us surfers and we used to call ourselves the Drops Crew. We were the opposite of hardcore.

There was Sorenson and Davey from the team and another VW enthusiast from Newcastle called Ollie Wickham. We'd travel up and down the coast in my Kombi, looking for a surf and putting some soup on the Primus. The furthest we went up the coast was to Thurso on the north coast of Scotland. What an amazing place. A beautiful beach, and in the summer, it basically never got dark. There'd be deer wandering across the road to the beach, so they obviously didn't feel under much shooting pressure.

About the only thing about Newcastle I didn't embrace was the local drop, Newcastle Brown Ale. I wasn't a fan, and no matter how hard the locals tried to convince me, it stayed that way. Looking at me now, I wish there were a lot more drinks that I found as repellent as the 'Broun Ale'.

In my final year at Newcastle, I was captain. I was enjoying the rugby. It was a better standard than club rugby in New Zealand, obviously, but there were parts of it that felt similar. There was no segregation at Newcastle between the supporters and the players. We'd often head to the supporters' club after a home game and drink and mix with the fans. I enjoyed that aspect. It was a neat part of English rugby.

I was hoping my third season at the club would be a take-off point, but if anything we went backwards. Again, we were left in a position where avoiding relegation was our only realistic ambition. As much as I was enjoying my footy, our results were not what the club wanted.

My contract was coming to an end, and I had a choice to make. We had investigated going to Johannesburg and I started to wonder whether playing Super Rugby, even in South Africa, would enable me still to be available for the All Blacks. Nat wasn't really that keen on the idea of living in South Africa, so we nixed that idea.

I did think about extending my stay at Newcastle. I was a reasonably loyal sort of bloke and there was part of me that wanted to finish the project I'd started to make Newcastle a force, but there seemed to be too many things happening off the field, including the constant turnover in coaches, that would always get in the way. We'd made progress in a few areas, including not being easybeats on the road, but I would have been lying to myself if I thought we'd done anything other than tread water for the three seasons I was there. The play-offs remained elusive.

I had two attractive options: Toulon, who had expressed an interest in me, or return to New Zealand.

I was really honest about the New Zealand situation, stating that I only wanted to come back for 12 months, play a Super Rugby season and be eligible for selection for the home World Cup, which was a tantalising prospect if I was good enough. If I wasn't good enough, I'd head back overseas. NZR were pretty adamant that they wanted a two- to three-year deal, and the simple fact was I didn't want to commit to an extended stay. It frustrated me and it only got worse when somebody forwarded me an article quoting Hurricanes CEO Greg Peters, who was saying NZR would get their pound of flesh from Hayman, or words to that effect.

I didn't read a lot of media but this article, in the *Sunday Star-Times*, really got me worked up. All the residual resentments I had towards the way I left New Zealand came to the surface again.

The *Sunday Star-Times* has learnt the giant prop is now sold on the idea of coming home from England to finish his career, if his terms can be met. And that has sparked a flurry of activity in the Wellington business community, with Hurricanes boss Greg Peters trying to solicit third-party funding to help Hayman realise his dream of buying a farm in Taranaki.

The New Zealand Rugby Union has moved heaven and earth to get Hayman home in time for the 2011 World Cup, digging deep to fund the majority of his considerable salary. But it is about $150,000 short, so the Hurricanes have been brought in on the deal and have been asked if they can cover the shortfall by exploring avenues such as third-party funding.

Peters said a 'number of parties were interested' in helping secure Hayman's signature, and it was vital the Wellington and New Zealand rugby unions worked together with the private business sector to get the deal done.

'Taranaki would be first port of call [for the NPC],'
Peters said. 'But we would love to see him playing for the
Hurricanes.'

This was before anything was even close to being signed. I was
sitting there like: 'Where is this shit coming from? Who is
leaking these talks?'

I'd made it crystal clear I only wanted to come back for a year
before going back overseas. If that didn't suit NZR's contracting
philosophy, so be it. I wasn't going to cry about it, because I had
options that were going to help set up my family for life.

But reading this sort of stuff brought the memories flooding
back about NZR buying me a farm and I was left with this
horrible feeling that I was involved in bad-faith negotiations
again. At the same time, a different, far more positive set of
memories also came to me, that of the van tour that Nat and I
took through France.

I started to look more closely at Toulon, a team on the
Mediterranean coast of France, who were building towards
something pretty special, having made the final of the second-
tier European Challenge Cup and the semi-finals of the
French Top 14 the previous season. Jonny Wilkinson had left
Newcastle to go there, Tana Umaga was there (although he
was about to leave), and the stars seemed to be aligning.

The only thing I had to wrestle with was forgoing the
opportunity to play a World Cup on home soil. But then again,

even if I went home, there was no guarantee that my game was still going to be what Ted was looking for. Owen Franks was a strong young man and it wasn't like he was just going to hand the No. 3 jersey back.

It's probably the right time to say I've never agreed with the rule that says you can't pick overseas-based players for the All Blacks, but then again, I probably would say that. At one point, I was advised by a couple of people (whom I won't name) that I should be the spearhead for a legal challenge to that ruling, and although it would have been a fascinating case, I had no interest in being the rocker of that particular boat. I'd made my career decisions with my eyes wide open, and just because I didn't agree with the 'rules', I knew what they were when I signed. While the common consensus is that by opening up selection, you'd have a mass exodus of good players leaving New Zealand for the big-money leagues in France, England and Japan, it's probably not realistic. European clubs in particular would not be interested in paying top dollar for a player they would have only limited access to. One of the reasons I was paid so handsomely was that once I was there, the clubs knew they had me, barring injury, for the entire season. Clubs would be far less willing to pay top dollar for an All Black who could be missing for large chunks of the season.

Ultimately Nat and I made the decision to move to Toulon. I knew my career with the All Blacks was finished for good, but there was no real sadness on my part. I'd actually come to the conclusion that it wasn't worth the trouble, as the obsession with what I was going to do next and what it was going to cost was getting on my nerves. I could almost hear the commentary the first time I dropped the ball or went backwards in a scrum: 'We bought this bloke a farm for *that*?'

As it was, when my signing for Toulon was announced, money was, of course, on the top of the agenda for the press. This from the *New Zealand Herald*.

Details of the fabulous financial rewards for Carl Hayman to give up on his dream of returning to New Zealand to help the All Blacks win the 2011 World Cup were emerging last night.

Sources at French Top 14 club Toulon say the former All Black, regarded as the No. 1 tighthead prop in world rugby, has negotiated a deal potentially worth over €1.86 million ($3.5 million).

The deal is believed to be for two years, with a further one year's option.

But the salary, €620,000 ($1.2 million) per season, is a formidable amount of money that raises the bar worldwide on the value of the best rugby players around the globe.

Revelations of Hayman's salary will bring broad smiles to the faces of Tri Nations players such as Daniel

Carter, Richie McCaw, Matt Giteau, Victor Matfield and others who may be thinking of moving to the Northern Hemisphere once the World Cup is over by the end of next year.

It might have brought broad smiles to their faces. This sort of story only brought a grimace to mine.

11

TAUPŌ, 2020, IRON MAN

I MIGHT HAVE BEEN five years removed from my playing career, but I was still a sucker for the thrill of the crowd.

The relief of unclipping myself from the pedals, getting out of the saddle and replacing that with the simplicity of a pair of running shoes was liberating enough, but when you combined it with the cheering of the crowd that lined the lakefront esplanade of Taupō, it was a heady mixture.

After a combined seven and a half hours in the water and six on the bike, it felt like just what I needed. A few people recognised me from my rugby days. Hearing people call your name and appreciate you no matter how far back in the field you were was gratifying. My fatigue just melted away.

What I didn't count on was that the feeling was fleeting. Suddenly, you realise the crowds have thinned out, you're pretty much alone on the open road and that mental high gives way to physiological reality. You glance at your watch and see that you've been doing 5 minute 20 second kilometres — way too fast. I was at about 17 kilometres, still with 25 kilometres to go, when the wheels started to fall off. It dawns on you that no amount of people cheering you on is going to get you to that finish line. It's your legs, your heart and your own mind that are going to have to do the heavy lifting there. What you have to do then is put the kilometre count out of your mind and focus on getting from aid station to aid station. You know you're going to have food and drink there and you can get enough fuel in to get to the next one, and so on. That's pretty much how I dragged myself to the finish line in 2020.

Welcome to the mindwarp that is an Ironman triathlon.

* * *

You can trace my entry into the world of endurance events back to a charity bike ride I did in 2019 for the My Name'5 Doddie Foundation. Doddie Weir is a former Scotland lock — hence the No. 5 in the name of the foundation — whom I got to know during my time at Newcastle. He was in charge of corporate events and was on the PA on match days. He was a fantastic MC and public speaker. In 2017, he announced that he had been diagnosed with motor neurone disease, a particularly cruel neurodegenerative disease that causes the loss of motor neurons that control muscles. As it progresses, it can affect your speech. A big part of Doddie's charm had always been his ability to communicate with all comers. For him to be robbed of that ability is a brutal example of how unfair life can be.

Doddie died in November 2022, just weeks after appearing at Murrayfield, where he delivered the match ball for the Scotland–New Zealand Test onto the field in his wheelchair.

There is a link between MND and CTE. A recent study of former Scottish rugby players determined that they were 15 times more likely to get MND than the general population. Some of those whose brains were studied post-mortem were found to have not only CTE, but the early signs of MND as well. It's an area where we still have so much to learn.

The charity ride was from John o' Groats at the top of Scotland to Land's End in Cornwall via London. A mutual friend asked me if I wanted to ride a few stages. I was out of work at the time so had no reason not to, apart from the fact I hadn't really ridden a road bike before. I got to John o' Groats with a borrowed bike, clipped in and rode 100 metres down the road and back just to make sure I could clip in and out without damaging myself or the bike and that was it. That was my preparation.

In the end, I ended up doing the whole ride and spent the first four days through Scotland thinking my life was about to end. My knees and neck were killing me, not to mention my backside. My arms were hanging like dead weights. We were doing between 140 and 180 kilometres a day of pack cycling. There were five of us who stayed the whole' course. Iwan Tukalo, the Scotland wing, who played a lot with Doddie, was one, as was Bryan Redpath, who played 60 Tests for Scotland at halfback.

Later that year, I was going to Nepal to hang out in the mountains for six weeks. I carried on training on the bike in France, tackling some of the hill climbs that the Tour de France peloton rides in the Pyrenees and the Alps. One I took on was the Col du Tourmalet, the highest paved mountain pass in the French Pyrenees and one of the most famous climbs on the Tour. It has been included more than any other pass and the Vuelta a España, the third of the three Grand Tours alongside France and the Giro d'Italia, has also crossed the pass several times. The first rider over in Tour de France history was Octave Lapize, who went on to win in 1910. Up to 2020, the Tour has visited the Col du Tourmalet close to 90 times, and since 1980, it has been ranked hors catégorie, or impossible to rate. Each summer, they move a large iron sculpture to the top of the climb. It's based on Lapize gasping for air as he struggles to make his way across the top of the pass, and I can testify to his struggles. I rode it on my mountain bike. In the Alps, I also rode across the Col du Petit-St-Bernard, which sits on the French–Italian border. It might not have the same historical and romantic cachet as the Tourmalet, but it's another brutal climb.

When I returned to New Zealand in 2019, I was determined to carry on with my fitness, so I worked towards a half Ironman in Taupō. When I completed that, I realised that if I were ever going to complete a full Ironman, this was the time to do it. I was fit and feeling good about myself, so I signed up there and then and committed to the Ironman in four months' time.

The process of preparing myself for an Ironman was revealing. I began to understand how rule-bound my life had been when I was a professional rugby player, and how that had been both a positive in terms of my discipline, and a negative when it came to intrinsic motivation — self-determination, I guess, and just the ability to think for myself. A big part of my mental health struggles when I retired, I believe, can be traced to the fact that the rugby training and timetable had pretty much been the only thing that gave my life a sharp focus. I didn't miss the games or the recovery, but the discipline and clarity I got from training left a far bigger hole in my life when it was gone than I had ever anticipated.

I wasn't hanging around rugby for the accolades, but I missed the feeling of a good training session, and I missed the structure; I missed having my week organised for me. I had that for 20 years. I knew where I had to be and what I had to do.

I also knew, for the most part, that it was good for me. When I stopped playing I stopped training altogether and that's when I felt my health starting to get away from me. I put on weight pretty quickly, and realised I needed to do something about it. When I started running again, the aches in my joints were close to unbearable. My knees felt like they wanted to fall off.

That initial stage was tough to get through, with the blisters and the aches and pains, the getting used to staring at a black line on the bottom of a pool. But Ironman got me back into familiar mental territory, with a fairly rigid training timetable built into my week.

Long-term, I don't think it will be physically sustainable for me to train for Ironman. The 70.3 events are probably more realistic, with my aching knees and back. But for the last three or four years, it's been a positive thing to get into and a great way to meet new people. It's also nice to go into a sport where there is no expectation on me to do well. I'm a big unit, but there are bigger people who do Ironmans. You'd be surprised. It's one of the great things about the sport. You get on the start line expecting to see nothing but sleek racehorse types, but it's actually all shapes and sizes and all athletic abilities. Some of the people, the recreational Ironmen and -women, are out on the course for 17 hours. They're literally competing against themselves and their own limitations for twice as long as the more natural athletes. It shows some serious ticker to be able to do that. How can you not respect the hell out of that achievement?

I took 12 hours 49 minutes for my first Ironman. I was thinking I could manage around 12 hours. My training, which I took from online advice, followed a broad outline but there was some ad libbing as well. The hardest thing for me to get my head around was the concept of long and slow. Coming from a rugby background where your training was tailored to short, explosive bursts, this messed with my mind a bit. The idea of running at seven-minute kilometres on a reasonably flat run, that was tough to compute. You think you're doing yourself a favour by running closer to six-minute kilometres, but you're not. You're actually making life tougher for yourself. With the help of a coach, Blair Cox, who was a Commonwealth Games cycling medallist and is big into the Ironman scene, I started to understand the physical mechanics, nutrition and exercise requirements of endurance sport. I understood how important the handbrake was when I was running, and although it might not have looked pretty if you were driving past — a 110-kilogram former prop chugging along at a speed barely above walking pace — I began to understand and enjoy the discipline required to do it.

It also got me thinking about my rugby career and how blasé I had been about certain aspects of it, particularly around in-game nutrition. All I'd take in during a game was a bit of electrolyte drink, but if I had my time again, I would start experimenting — perhaps a gel at 60 minutes or some superfoods at halftime. I'm sure players these days are far more scientific about what they take in, but when I was starting out, it was literally oranges at halftime and not too much water because you'd get the stitch. It initially felt weird to ingest so much food while training, but it's what you have to do in endurance events. On long bike rides, you'd stop at a bakery and have a pie and a can of Coke and it was great: no guilt at all.

I might have had ambitions to break the 12-hour mark in my first Ironman, but as I got deeper into the race, I realised it was more about health, wellbeing, fitness and, crucially, finishing. The time was irrelevant. It got me out the door doing something positive. I've never met anybody who has felt mentally worse after a good training session.

Of the three triathlon disciplines, I enjoy running the most, but I also realise it's the worst for my joints. It's the simplicity and convenience of it that appeals to me. If you find yourself with a spare half-hour, just slip your shoes on and head out for a trot. Biking requires a bit more organisation, a lot more cost and is not much fun on busy city streets and roads. It's much better on my knees and hips. I have to admit, I don't really like swimming. Even though the outdoor pool at New Plymouth's public baths is a beautiful venue, the monotony of staring at the bottom of the pool gets to you pretty quickly. I try to get at least one open-water swim in each week — not too difficult when my place sits on the edge of Port Taranaki and Ngāmotu Beach.

I crossed the line a little more than half an hour quicker at my second Ironman, again at Taupō. Like my first attempt, I got into a dark place on the run. You get out past the fire station and people slowly disappear. There are no supporters and the reality slowly sinks in: I'm on my own here and there is a long way to go. This time it happened much further down the course.

The second time around I was really happy with my run. I was on course for a sub-four-hour marathon, averaging a little more than 10 km/h up to the 30-kilometre mark but I should have known that nothing comes easy in this sport. With about 10 kilometres to go I started to tie up. It wasn't a full-blown physical breakdown, but I knew my tanks were close to empty. That last section took more than 90 minutes to complete.

There's no feeling quite like the last few hundred metres of an Ironman. You can't compare it to the thrill of victory in a rugby match. That's a shared moment with mates and the satisfaction of doing your jobs better than the opposition. It's a great feeling, don't get me wrong, but there's something almost spiritual about completing an endurance event. When I came down the red carpet at the end of my first Ironman, I was emotional in a way I had never experienced with rugby. There were definitely tears welling up. You spend a lot of the day thinking about that moment while all the time wondering if your body is capable of getting you there. In my case, I had never even run a marathon, but here I was tacking one on to the end of a long, cold-water swim and a 180-kilometre bike ride. A sense of satisfaction didn't come close to summing it up.

I had to be brutally honest and say I hadn't done a lot to be proud of since my playing career had ended, but this was an achievement I could grasp on to and say I did something that I never knew I was capable of; that I did it largely on my own and I made myself better physically and mentally in the process.

With my condition, I don't know what the future holds and I don't know whether the longer endurance events are going to continue to be feasible. I'm the sort of guy who needs goals to work towards, so if it's not Ironman events, it will have to be something else.

Staying fit can only be a good thing. It has to be a non-negotiable part of my future.

2020: Swim 1h 15m 28s; Bike 6h 17m; Run 4h 51m 13s.
Total: 12h 49m 07s

2021: Swim 1h 16m 47s; Bike 6h 30 50s; Run 4h 26m 42s.
Total: 12h 26m 04s

12

TOULON, 2010–15, BREAK POINT

WHILE YOU MIGHT BE able to trace my cognitive decline to the moment I picked up an oval ball and ran with it, I pinpoint my time at Toulon as the moment it started to come into a jarring, fuzzy type of focus.

The irony, if that's the correct way to describe it, is that if I had any glory years as a rugby player, the bulk of them happened while playing for this awakened giant of European rugby. After a rocky start, Rugby Club Toulonnais embraced me, and I embraced the club. The city, arguably the least glamorous town on the French Riviera, was made for me. It breathed rugby through its pores. I loved representing the people and the city.

But the rugby was brutal, relentless. Playing with pain was not just accepted, but expected. If it took an unhealthy cocktail of painkillers and, yes, alcohol, to get me through to another match day, that's what I did.

My status at Toulon went on a sharp upwards trajectory as my health plummeted. That's hindsight. I didn't really see it at the time. It's only when you step away with some distance that you start to understand the warning signs that were missed — the stabbing headaches, the constant pain, the frequent disorientation and spells of déjà vu, the increased reliance on alcohol for sleep, the mood swings — but at the time you convinced yourself this was part and parcel of pro rugby. If I'm feeling like this, others must be, too, right?

There's a perverse pleasure to be had in it. If it took all my willpower to drag my carcass out of bed the morning after a game because my back and neck were screaming at me to stay prone, that just meant I'd done my job. You justified it by saying that everyone at the club, everyone in professional rugby, was feeling the same things to an extent — and if your extent was greater than others', then that was something to take pride in, to celebrate, because it just made you that much tougher.

It meant a lot to me to be tougher than most. It justified my wage. It justified my elevation to captaincy. It was an intrinsic part of Carl Hayman, the brand. Yeah, I might cringe at that now, as I flub away large chunks of days in New Plymouth in a dull fog, struggling to remember the task I was doing 10 minutes ago and desperately searching for reasons to be cheerful, but back then, it was a different story.

I was someone to be respected. Maybe even a little bit feared.

I was peak 'Carl Hayman' at Toulon. I had no idea how ephemeral that peak would be and how slippery the slope on the other side was.

It was my high point.

It was where I started to fall.

* * *

I met the inimitable Toulon owner and comic-book millionaire Mourad Boudjellal in Paris before I signed for his club. I dined with him at the Gare du Nord, the terminus for the Eurostar that links France and Britain via the Channel Tunnel and the busiest train station in Europe. We had lunch at Terminus Nord, a grand old white-tablecloth restaurant within the station. It was pretty fancy for a bloke brought up on a dairy farm.

We met with my player agent, Laurent Lafitte. In my mind, Laurent was the quintessential Frenchman, very smooth, slick hair, a great talker with a heavy accent. All he was missing was the beret and ubiquitous baguette under his arm to himself be a comic-book character. Laurent had most of the New Zealand-born players on his books through what was then Essentially, but is now Halo Sports, my management company. By law, you needed a French agent to play in France.

Mourad didn't really need to reach into his bag of hard-sell tricks. It wouldn't have mattered how good the filet de boeuf was. Something drew me to Toulon. Yes, the money was good, and it would be stupid to try to deny that it played a part, especially knowing this was probably my last big contract, but it was far from the only reason. It probably wasn't even the main reason, although it's easy to say that now. That trip Nat and I had taken in the Kombi van during my first northern summer was the hard sell, and a morning croissant was the currency. I knew nothing about Toulon, but I knew it was in France, and that was all that mattered.

The first time I set foot in the city was the day I moved there. The Newcastle season finished at the start of May and we weren't meeting for pre-season until the middle of June, so I made a pledge to myself to get really fit. I was training every day by myself. I'd head out for long runs around Newcastle and its surrounds. I'd go to the gym and push big weights. I was feeling pretty good about myself when I landed at Nice Airport.

What I didn't expect was a reception committee. I suddenly realised what it must feel like to be Dan Carter. As I entered the arrivals hall, there were reporters, photographers and even Mourad was there to greet me. There's that uncomfortable feeling where you know they're probably there for you, but you don't want to look like a dick and present yourself just in case Jonny Wilkinson is arriving at the same time and the camera operators walk straight past you.

I needn't have worried. It was me they were there for, after all. It dawned on me how revered the scrum is in France. There's a saying: 'No scrum, no win', and they live by it. You can have a really poor game and lose, but if you dominate their scrum, you're the toast of the town. You compare that to the way New Zealanders view the game. They'd say there was no point in having a good set piece if you were losing and that we needed to shift the ball out of those tight areas. In France, the idea that there could be 'no point' in having a good scrum went against everything they believed in.

Those early days were fairly difficult. I wished I'd taken more time to learn the language, because I was literally starting out with 'bonjour' and 'merci' as the only words I knew. While you can get away without learning the language in a rugby environment — English was a default that most of the French people could speak, even if they'd rather not — I decided it would be a travesty to spend three years in the country and not learn how to at least have basic conversations with the locals. Natalie did a language course at the local polytech and I did my lessons through the club. Nat probably got more out of her course than I did out of mine. A friend of mine was the teacher, and so if you can imagine a school holiday programme where the kids get to play outside most of the day but are forced to do an hour of lessons inside where they spend it throwing paper darts at the teacher, that's what our classes were like. There were some of us who were interested in learning, but others would try to sidetrack the teacher into explaining unnecessary stuff so they wouldn't have to get their books out. Fortunately, I ended up becoming good friends with a French-language teacher and it really unlocked some doors in terms of experiencing a true Gallic lifestyle.

Toulon is an interesting town. It's a big naval and armaments city, so much of the port area is a militarised zone. It's not renowned as one of the more attractive cities on the Côte d'Azur, but it has its own charms. If you're after glamour, however, you'll find more to the east in nearby St Tropez, Cannes, Nice and Monaco.

What was really special about playing for Toulon is that the stadium, Stade Félix Mayol, usually just known as Stade Mayol, is slap-bang in the middle of the city, down by the port. With all the nearby bars and restaurants, the game-day atmosphere is always fantastic. For French rugby supporters, regardless of what team they follow, going and watching a game in Toulon was a highlight of the season. The ground is legendary for its passionate crowd. There's a saying that roughly translates to 'the wind blows too strong through the locals' hair and makes them crazy'.

Toulon has some nice parts to it, but during the war a lot of the city was bombed because of the naval base. The town was rebuilt but there's a real contrast between the nice old parts that were untouched and the more functional, less attractive rebuilt parts. Nat and I bought a place in Carqueiranne, a little fishing village about 20 minutes' drive east of the city. Even after the games, we didn't spend that much time in the city itself. Conveniently, the training centre was on the northeastern outskirts of Toulon as well, so there was no need to drive all the way into town from Carqueiranne for practices.

What was a nice contrast to Newcastle was that this was unquestionably a rugby town. In Newcastle all the chatter was football, football, football, with just a smattering of rugby. Here it was the complete opposite. It was all rugby. People loved their rugby team. If they bothered to talk about football, it was usually about the fortunes of Olympique Marseille, the nearest Ligue 1 football club.

A lot of the smaller, traditional rugby towns like Béziers and Clermont might argue, but Toulon — or Rugby Club Toulonnaise, to give it the proper name — is renowned for having the most fanatical supporters. The coach when I got there, Philippe Saint-André, used to talk about how if we won, the supporters in Toulon would treat us like gods, but if we lost, they'd quickly go the other way.

The forwards coach was former Les Bleus halfback Aubin Hueber, who used to always say that in France it is the scrumhalf who knows the scrums. I'd never known any halfback that knew a great deal about scrums, so that got my alarm bells ringing. It turned out that Hueber was a very good talker, but I'm more convinced than ever that halfbacks know fuck-all about scrums. So, yeah, that's as good an indication as any that my first year at Toulon was difficult, like it was in Newcastle, but for a different reason. I didn't end up playing anywhere near as much as I should have.

It was awkward, because there was a lot of hype around my arrival. I'd appeared on all these media grabs and promos about how much I was looking forward to the Top 14 and there were all these French props out there, thinking: 'Yeah, we'll show the Kiwi big-noter how much he should be looking forward to it.' They were licking their chops a bit. 'Bienvenue en France, trou du cul — welcome to France, asshole!'

Like Newcastle, it took me a bit of time to fit in and build relationships with the guys I was playing with, like hooker Seb Bruno and loosehead Laurent Emmanuelli. The Georgian tighthead Davit Kubriashvili was often preferred. He was a strong young guy, and I didn't begrudge him his opportunities or success. But you couldn't hide the fact I was being paid big money for the job he was doing.

The refereeing around scrums was completely different in France, as was the way they actually scrummed. It seemed so imbalanced compared to what I was used to. My calling card was speed across the middle on the call of 'engage' — a skill that has been taken out of the game with the way the scrums are packed down now. That, and knowing how to keep our scrum stable and balanced from which we could work strike moves. In France, they thrived more on chaos, on creating imbalances and winning penalties. That wasn't my game, but I knew I'd have to learn it pretty quickly, or else I was going to be a massive waste of money. Mourad was never slow to let the public know when he thought he was throwing good money after bad. Just ask All Black wing Julian Savea. In 2019, Boudjellal said: 'I'm going to ask for a DNA test. They must have swapped him on the plane. If I were him, I would apologise and go back to my home country.'

Boudjellal never said the same thing about me — not to my face, anyway — but I did hear that he was keen on asking key people at the club: 'Where's the Carl Hayman we used to see on TV?'

Ouch.

I had ideas on how to improve the situation, especially in the scrums, but as a foreigner in my first year, my suggestions were not met with open arms. Quite the opposite, if I'm being truthful. I'm a shy guy as a rule, and it would take quite a bit for me to push myself forward, especially in a language I was grappling with. In not so many words, I was countered with an attitude of: 'Hey, this is France. You'll do things our way.' That would make me want to shrink into the background even more.

It was hugely frustrating and perhaps even a little bit embarrassing because if I wasn't the best-paid player at the club, then I was right up there and I had two choices: keep pushing my ideas and potentially alienate my coaches and teammates; or sit back, shut up, take the hits to my ego by not playing regularly and try to learn a new and, in my opinion, inferior way of operating.

In that first season, I mostly, but not always, shut up and tried to see the positive side of it. I'd played so many seasons in a row with the volume turned up to maximum. On the one hand, my being on the outer at Toulon gave me an unscheduled opportunity to recharge, to train well and to fix a few niggles. I was still being paid and I had a fixed contract, so even in a worst-case scenario — being frozen out — I was still going a long way to setting up the family's future. On the other hand, I couldn't help but wonder if I would have been better off taking up the opportunity in New Zealand and playing in a home World Cup.

I was still playing games off the bench, but when it came to the Heineken Cup quarter-final loss to Perpignan in Barcelona, I wasn't even involved in the match-day squad. That might have had something to do with a recent incident where my frustrations with Aubin had come to a head. He liked to come out and do warm-ups and run around with the reserves as a halfback and do a bit of work with the defence. One day, I saw an opportunity. I saw him at the base of a ruck. I felt like a bull in an arena where the matador loses his concentration for a second and I just went through and cleaned him out right through this ruck. There was a lot of pent-up frustration in the act. It was a bit of a cheap shot, but shit, it felt good. Having said that, there was a fair chunk of the season left and I didn't play much of the rest of it, so who do you reckon won that battle of wills? I'll give you a clue: it wasn't me.

My woes were not all Aubin's fault. While I was really fit that season — my aerobic capacity was probably as good as it's ever been — I was tipping the scales at 117–118 kilograms, and I was probably just too light for French rugby. It was such an abrasive, contact-dominant game. I was getting through games and still had heaps to give in the legs and the lungs. I was covering ground almost like a loose forward, but that wasn't what they had signed me on to do. They'd signed me to be a monster in the scrum and brutal at the ruck and maul — nothing that would have a positive effect on my brain, obviously, but I wasn't to know that then. In the off-season, I went away and put some more muscle on the frame —no more cells in the brain, unfortunately — and the next year I came back at an imposing 122 kilograms.

I was 30 years old, supposedly entering my peak years as a prop, and right from the word go, it was a different ball game. Philippe Saint-André was still there, though he was promoted to France coach halfway through the season, but Olivier Azam, a hooker who could play prop and who had just retired from playing, had taken over from Aubin as forwards coach. Azam was French but spent most of his career at Gloucester, so his

English was excellent and he came in with a clean slate. He probably won't mind me saying this, but he was a dirty bugger on the field. I played against him for Newcastle and it wasn't a lot of fun — he'd mouth off, throw in a bit of trash talk and had this habit of standing on your hands whenever he got the chance. Despite all that, I was looking forward to working with him because, well, he wasn't Aubin.

Before the season started, Olivier pulled me aside and told me he wanted me involved with a lot of the planning and work the coaches were doing, which was what I needed to hear after being frozen out the previous season. You'd think in my thirties I wouldn't need that kind of reassurance, but it gave my confidence a boost when it was threatening to sag.

We still needed some stability in the playing roster — Toulon was always in such a rush to find success that players would come and go at an unsustainable rate — but after finishing with a 15–11 record and an eighth place in 2010–11, missing the play-offs in the process, things were heading in a positive direction for me and the team. We had a number of high-profile recruits, like Bakkies Botha, Matt Giteau and later Drew Mitchell, and they were all signings to add value in specific areas we needed, not just vanity signings for Mourad or panic buys when things weren't going well.

Our strength and conditioning trainer was a guy called Steve Walsh. I give him a lot of credit for keeping me strong and (kind of) injury-free deep into my thirties. Walsh was a sharp-tongued North Englishman who had a league background, having worked with Wigan and then Leeds before switching codes to Sale. He was headhunted by Philippe in 2009 and was given free licence to build an athletic performance facility to his own specifications. By general agreement, what he built for us at Toulon was miles ahead of any other club. We had the usual free weights and cardio machines, but there was also a five-lane 30 metre running track of double thickness for plyometrics, four six-metre ropes hanging from the ceiling and two machines that were purely focused on building strength and flexibility into the hamstring and gluteal muscles. Steve had analysed the type of injuries that kept rugby players out for the most time and realised upper leg muscles were a killer. The machines were supposedly based on designs used by coaches of Communist-era East European gymnasts. There was a sadistic side to Steve, so it wouldn't have surprised me.

Steve had an uncanny sense of knowing when the older guys like me and Bakkies Botha needed a hard session and when we just needed to get on the foam rollers. That could cause a few problems with the younger academy guys, who saw what these older, high-priced players were getting away with, but Steve had the force of personality to push it through.

Another new recruit in my second year at the club was Andy Sheridan, a powerful loosehead prop from England. When you put me, Seb Bruno and Andy in the same front row, on paper, at least, it was pretty formidable. It was also tall. I came in at 1.93 metres and Andy was 1.95 metres. Poor old Seb must have felt like a Lilliputian trapped between two Gullivers as he stretched himself out to his fullest at 1.74 metres.

Andy didn't take long to establish a name for himself as a destructive loosehead. If you look at his Wikipedia page, there's an interesting section about his first Test for England:

In England's November Test against Australia, [Sheridan played] the main role in outclassing the Australian front row. Neither of his opposite numbers finished the match. First, Al Baxter proved unable to deal with Sheridan's power, and was eventually sin-binned late in the second half for collapsing a scrum after being warned for repeated scrum violations. Shortly afterwards, Matt Dunning, who was forced to move opposite Sheridan, was stretchered off after a scrum with what was feared to be a serious neck injury; however, scans showed no structural damage to his neck. Due to the sin-binning and Dunning's injury, the referee ordered uncontested scrums for the last 10 minutes of the match. He faced Carl Hayman of the All Blacks the next Saturday, who gave him a tough time at the scrum by scrumming very low, negating Sheridan's raw power.

I'd had some great tussles with Andy in Test rugby and also when Newcastle played Sale. In most respects, we were quite different people, but we did share a common trait, in that we liked to be left alone to get on with our jobs. Andy was a big lifter in the gym. He loved throwing tin around. He was a freak. I thought I was keen on the gym, but I'd never come across anybody like him. He'd take himself and a spotter down to the far end of the room, away from the noise, and away he'd go, lifting incredible weights. He could bench-press 235 kilograms and squat 275, which puts him in elite powerlifting company.

The new signings, the familiarity with my teammates and the arrival of Bernard Laporte — the architect of the All Blacks' demise in 2007 — as coach and the knowledge that this was going to be the last significant contract of my career, were the catalysts for some of my best rugby memories as my three-year contract stretched out to five.

I was starting to get to grips with some of the cultural nuances in French rugby that had baffled me in season one. One of those is the real home-and-away mentality. The attitude among French players was borderline defeatist before away games, even if you were playing less talented teams. If we lost on the road, there was this clichéd, Gallic, c'est la vie shrug of the shoulders. 'Never mind. We'll get them when they come to Toulon later in the season,' was the common refrain. Get those same players, so blasé on the road, on home turf and they would play like lions defending their cubs. A lot of energy was expended before home games talking about defending your territory and doing it for your people. For an outsider, especially one who played for the All Blacks where every away Test was seen as an opportunity to execute what we practised and impose our way of playing on the home team, the whole thing was a bit weird. How many times can you get psyched up by the principal motivation of 'defending your citadel'? The French never seemed to tire of it. They'd leave the darkness of the changing rooms and run into the sunlight of the Stade Mayol 10 feet tall and breathing fire out of their noses. When you play on high emotion, it becomes harder and harder to replicate that every week, so you save it for 'your people' and dial it back when playing away from home. That's a generalised way of looking at it, but I noticed it with the coaching as well. In my experience, the French coaches tugged on those emotional levers far more than English-speaking coaches, who were more systems- and detail-oriented.

That attitude can't help but seep into what you do, no matter how limited you believed this approach to rugby was. I'd find myself playing right on the edge some weeks and feeling really flat the next. In New Zealand rugby, the best coaches like Ted, Shag and Smithy were big on players making 'blue-headed' decisions, which is really the ability to make calm, rational choices in the heat of battle. In France, they love to play with a 'red' head, and the crowd feeds off that emotion, too. Sure, it can be a potent weapon, but it can also be counterproductive when things aren't going your way.

Even if we had the most clear-headed mandate, dialled back on the emotion and played picture-perfect training-ground rugby, winning away would still be difficult in France. It's hard to explain why without getting too mystical, but there's just an energy from the crowd that's hard to overcome, for referees too. I'm not sure if there are any accurate stats for this, but 50–50 calls tend to go with the home team more in France than anywhere else I've played.

Toulon were especially unloved on the road. We had a lot of foreign players and there was a real edge — hostility even — from the away crowds. We were seen as the club for mercenaries and, for a long period there, the team every other side most badly wanted to beat. At Clermont Auvergne, where Vern Cotter coached for many years, it wasn't unusual for their supporters to throw stuff at our bus as we arrived.

I enjoyed it, even at its most overwhelming. It was quite something to hear the cheers and jeers and the band strike up in the stand if we conceded a scrum penalty, for example. In New Zealand, the crowd would probably be pissed off that the ref has found a technical infringement in the scrum and the game has stopped again, but in France, it was a crucial moral victory. I've played in games where we've won pretty comfortably and the other team's loosehead prop is fêted like an all-conquering hero after the game because he's trapped me into giving away a penalty or has forced a messy scrum. It surprised me at first, but you quickly learn to take your lumps and move on.

That home-ground mentality was at its peak when clubs from smaller southern cities like Béziers, Tarbes, Dax, Pau, Mont-de-Marsan, Perpignan and Castres among others were fighting not just for wins, but also for civic pride. I'm not saying that teams from Paris — Stade Français and Racing Metro — and the other big cities didn't play with the same pride, but there wasn't the same edge. You lose a big game for Racing, you can walk freely around Paris the next day; you lose a big game for Béziers (who play mainly in the second division, these days) and the whole town wants a piece of you for the next week.

Even so, the passion has been toned down somewhat. Talk to some of the old-timers about playing in the 1970s, '80s and '90s — back when guys like Jérôme Gallion, Marc de Rougement, Eric Melville and the legendary hard man Eric Champ were playing for Toulon — and it sounded like the wild west. That side of the game had been cleaned up in the professional ranks, but the wildest brawl I saw was when I was a player-coach at an amateur side in Pau, Avenir Bizanos, and there was a 30-man brawl that involved the crowd. I was sitting there, thinking: 'Shit, if this was in New Zealand, that's on the national news tonight.' I don't think it even warranted a mention in the local paper.

The actual violence had largely been regulated by the time I arrived. I experienced more eye-gouging and testicle-grabbing playing the French national team than I ever did in club rugby.

Widespread television coverage had put paid to the days of the all-in brawls that were commonplace, and the geography of French rugby was changing from the amateur days, too.

My second season at Toulon went a lot better. The short story is we won three Heineken Cups in a row, an unprecedented feat, and a Top 14 title in the 2013–14 season. Leinster, Leicester and Saracens have all won two on the bounce, but that Toulon side under Laporte remains the only team to win three.

The first title was an epic, beating Cotter's Clermont 16–15 in the final in Dublin. I don't care what anybody says, Clermont were better than us that day and scored two tries to one, but Jonny Wilkinson had a flawless day with the boot and Morgan Parra, the French halfback, missed one conversion and that was the difference.

Both teams had a Kiwi flavour. As well as Cotter the coach, they had Sitiveni Sivivatu and Regan King, brother of squash champion Joelle, and we had myself, Chris Masoe, and wings David Smith and Rudi Wulf.

The following season we were probably at our peak. In the Heineken Cup play-offs, we beat Irish giants Leinster and Munster before thrashing Saracens 23–6 in the final at Cardiff's Millennium Stadium. There's a nice photo of Jonny Wilkinson and me clutching the boxes that held our winners' medals, walking around Millennium Stadium in our Toulon uniforms that look more like billboards than footy jerseys, advertising VW and Orangina, among other things. I don't know what we're saying to each other, but our wide smiles tell the story.

A week after that final, we returned home to meet Castres in the final of the Top 14. In his final match, Jonny kicked 15 points and we won 18–10. The crowd at Stade de France, both sets of supporters, sang 'God Save the Queen' for him. I was bloody pleased for my little mate. Our band might never have become the chart-toppers we dreamed of, and we couldn't quite turn the Newcastle Falcons into the force we'd hoped to, but we did okay in the south of France together.

In those five do-or-die matches, including the Top 14 semi-final that we won against Racing Metro, no team came within a converted try of us. We simply bullied our way to the double.

In my final season, I was named captain to replace Jonny, a real honour. We topped the Top 14 table again, but were blown out in our semi-final against Stade Français, removing any hope of a double-double. We fared better in Europe, in the renamed Champions Cup, beating Clermont at Twickenham, a replay of the 2013 final, although we were a little more comfortable this time, winning 24–18, with Wales fullback Leigh Halfpenny, who had a howitzer-strength leg, scoring 14 points.

Yes, that's the short story, of games played and matches won. Of the glory, the post-final parades through Toulon, of that feeling that you have the freedom of the city.

It's the story I would have told in far greater detail had my book been penned in the immediate afterglow of my playing career. I loved Toulon and, by the end at least, even if the place didn't love me back, the team's fans held me in some sort of affection, I think.

But there's an element of that story which is a lie. A glorious lie, but a lie all the same. Toulon broke me. I was a willing participant, but I've come to realise that while the glory is fleeting, the damage is permanent.

I played 156 games for the club in five seasons, including the first when I didn't play as much as I anticipated. For most of my time there, we were fighting on two fronts: domestically, and in Europe. In France, even against the weaker teams, there is no such thing as an easy game for a prop. It was often a hard, physical, mentally sapping grind.

Pain was a constant. It came in different forms. It was nociceptive and neuropathic. It was throbbing, it was shooting. Sometimes it was localised; other times, my whole body felt like it had been through the wringer. Some pains would come and go, others hung around for the season, sometimes longer.

If you think about it, pain is a mere signal. It is a way for a part of your body to let the central nervous system know that something is wrong. As a rugby player, part of your job is to trick the central nervous system: to trick your own brain.

The most common way of doing this is through the administration of painkillers. Every rugby team I've played with has liberally used paracetamol and ibuprofen to dull the aches and pains, but in France, this was supercharged. Get any player who has played long enough there in a quiet, off-the-record moment and they'll tell you about whole seasons played alongside their best friends, tramadol and diclofenac (better known in New Zealand as Voltaren). They might also tell you about those long bus trips home, when team staff would move down the aisle with a portable medicine cabinet, dispensing pills like Skittles.

These pills became a clubhouse currency, like cigarettes in a prison or ecstasy at an all-night dance party. If you were really struggling with pain, this barter system allowed you to bypass the club medical staff to get what you needed to keep going. Because in European club rugby and in France in particular, keeping going was the name of the game. There was always another match around the corner, always another competition to win, always another scrum to pack down.

Sometimes I took injections and played. On one occasion, I had a nerve root injection in my cervical spine — the neck — during the week and was playing on the weekend. Playing with an inflamed nerve in your neck is pretty tricky as a prop. It's usually the result of an inflamed disc, the layer of cartilage that sits between the vertebrae. As you get older, your discs lose their water content and become harder and more compact. They lose their shock-absorbing qualities, and when you're using your neck as much as I did in my working life, they are susceptible to becoming inflamed and irritating the nerve that passes through them.

The injection made the pain bearable by reducing the inflammation, but it did nothing to address the structural damage to the discs. I've talked to physios about this since, and while they say it is possible to play a game of rugby just days after having one of these injections, to a person they said it would not have been 'in my best interests'.

Even though my best interests and the club's best interests diverge here, the greatest trick you play on yourself is to pretend they're the same. My ability to play through pain was never seen as stupid and misguided, a bad example to set for younger players. Instead, it was seen as necessary, as selfless and maybe even vaguely heroic. 'Look at Carl. He could be sitting on the sidelines cashing his cheques, but he's out there playing under extreme duress. Be like Carl.'

Painkillers might be a powerful drug, but not as powerful as that feeling that you're going above and beyond to help your team and your teammates. If I'd broken an arm or leg, it would have been easier, but my injuries — my badges of honour — didn't require casts or moon-boots. If I could stand up, I played, and I did that week after week after week for 10 months of the year for five years straight. I was, in effect, a useful slab of meat.

The amount of rugby we played was ridiculous but, again, when you're in the middle of it, you don't see as clearly. I was a professional rugby player, so it made all the sense in the world to keep playing. With the benefit of some distance from the game, I can see the insanity. When I first started playing professionally, I remember clearly going to a Players' Association meeting run by Rob Nichol and the primary point of concern raised was the need to establish a global window and having a shorter season. That was in the 1990s. Close to a quarter of the way through the twenty-first century and we're still having the same bloody conversations. It's too late for me, but we have to help protect the players of the present and future.

I've been quoted on this before, but it still rings true: look at the NFL season. That league is not without health problems, as has been well documented, but they have a 17-game season across four to five months with the possibility of a couple of play-off games. You compare that to rugby with a 10-month season and, if you're a strong club like Toulon, playing more than 30 games per season. Look at the All Blacks. They can play 13 or 14 Tests a year at the highest intensity and yet those same players are expected to play full seasons for their Super Rugby teams. It's ridiculous. There needs to be an urgent discussion about what constitutes an acceptable volume of rugby, because it's not what we see at the moment.

At the same time I was scaling the heights of European club rugby as a supposedly indestructible tighthead prop, I was falling apart, physically, mentally and emotionally.

I was starting to endure migraine headaches that started when I woke up in the morning and did not relent until I finally found sleep. I could largely keep up the front at my workplace, but at home I was in bits. My moods were all over the place.

There were these weird sensations creeping into the game. The best way I can describe it is déjà vu, where frequently I would experience the sensation of having been there in that exact moment before. But it was off the field where life was hardest. I was often forgetful and listless. I couldn't sleep and when I did, it was fitful and restless. My drinking at Toulon escalated from once-a-week binges to midweek drinking on my own.

Others around me saw the signs that all was not well, but I refused to acknowledge them or brushed them aside.

Everything would be all right once I retired and I could get on a farm and get some normality back in my life.

Wouldn't it?

13

NEW PLYMOUTH, 2022–23, STANDING UP

GATHERING MY THOUGHTS AND trying to put them in an ordered manner has been an invaluable experience, though it hasn't been easy. I'll be happy if this is an imperfect and, in parts, confused and confusing read because my life is confused and confusing. It's certainly imperfect.

In November 2022, just as the manuscript deadline for this book was approaching, I had an anxiety-induced, paranoid mental breakdown. It was not the impending deadline or the process of putting together the book that induced it. This has been a raw, but mostly cathartic experience. The meltdown was down to other causes altogether.

I'd been working on *Rescue III*, but I wasn't getting stuff done anywhere near as quickly and effectively as I should have. It started to gnaw away at me. Normally when this happens, I take a break and go into an unreachable zone. I might need to lie down or just sit there with a cup of tea staring out the window. Kiko spots it immediately. She knows that if I work too long or too hard, the energy in my brain depletes really quickly. It just leaves me zonked out and uncommunicative.

But summer was approaching, and I was getting really pissed off about how long this job was taking. It didn't matter how much help I was getting, including from my old Highlanders rugby flatmate Blair Feeney. Blair has been a godsend. He came to New Plymouth to stay and help me get *Rescue III* back on the water and, truth be told, to help Kiko keep an eye on me after a few previously mentioned setbacks. Blair's life has not been all chocolates and roses, either, so he recognises the pitfalls better than most.

I had a moment of the worst kind of clarity. It dawned on me that this was my life now — days that were speckled with momentary bursts of energy followed by long periods of physical and mental inertia. My days would start with a list of things that needed doing, a body that was built to do things and a broken mind that would not let it. And if this was my life now, what would it be like a year down the track, two years, five years?

That thought just filled me with so much anger and despair that I snapped. Those around me could see it coming. Things had been weighing more heavily on me since Mum died, but grief alone couldn't explain everything.

Everything I did felt so unstable. That's not figurative. Nothing felt balanced. Not my thought processes, not my emotional responses, not even my physical health. That instability and feeling of disorientation made me topple.

I left the shed and told Kiko I was done. I was done with the boat, I was done with the business and I was done with New Plymouth. I was moving to Ōpunake. I went off my antidepressant medication. I jumped in my truck and headed out of the city and down the coast. I did this all in a manic episode. There was no delay.

It was only once I reached the farm that the full-blown anxiety and panic attack hit, and I realised what I'd just done. I understood that on my own, isolated here on the farm, I wouldn't last long. I know 'last long' is a clumsy euphemism, but sometimes it's easier than saying your darkest thoughts out loud. But I must have said it out loud to Kiko, because pretty soon, a crisis team kicked into action. The right people gathered around me. I went back on my meds and things became clearer and calmer. Crisis momentarily averted.

There you go. I don't feel much better telling you this, but there's no point me writing about all the good and bad in my life if I'm not going to paint a true picture of where I'm at, what my day-to-day looks like, and why Kiko isn't just my best friend but sometimes much more than that, something she definitely didn't sign up for: my saviour.

* * *

We met on the charity bike ride from John o' Groats to Land's End. I'm going to put words in her mouth from time to time here, but we've talked about this often enough, so I think we've got our stories straight. She'll let me know if I haven't.

An important thing to note is that she vowed she would never go out with a rugby player, because they drank too much and were too lairy. There must be so many times she wished she'd taken her own advice.

When she was 28 and again at 36, Kiko had an aggressive form of Cushing's syndrome, a life-threatening condition she contracted as the result of a six-millimetre pituitary tumour. The syndrome carries with it a range of symptoms, including memory loss, muscle-wasting, osteoporosis, end-stage diabetes, insomnia and psychosis. During her first bout, Kiko's potassium levels dropped too low for her to risk the brain surgery necessary to remove the tumour, so she was forced into intensive care until she regained enough strength to survive the procedure.

She was acutely aware that life was short and was there to be grabbed.

So in 2018 she rowed solo across the Atlantic from La Gomera, one of Spain's Canary Islands, to Port St Charles in Barbados. It took her a tick over 49 days, which meant she broke the world record by a week. She also raised £105,000 for King's College Hospital in London, where she was treated, not knowing that one day she'd be back at the same place with her partner in tow, looking for answers about his brain.

We can be a bit blinkered in life, only bothering to understand what we know, so for most people rowing the Atlantic is either incomprehensible or their vision of hell. Kiko enjoyed it, despite getting sick, having to administer her own post-surgery medication — she'd had a second tumour removed just months before the row — and encountering rogue waves that could pitch you into the ocean without notice.

She got her name in some pretty prestigious publications after that feat, including ESPN, where a couple of things in her interview, which was given in the lead-up to her row across the Atlantic, resonate loudly today.

Capsizing in the middle of the night would be scary. But actually, if I think about it, I'm not fearful. Why do we fear death when we know the only thing that's certain in life is that we're not going to live forever?

You could have a day of lonely, painful drowning, but I'd rather that than have a slow, painful death over several years. It's totally a mental thing. It's training yourself to not worry. And I won't.

That's the difference between Kiko and me. All I do is worry about the future.

That goal ticked off, she was looking for two things: a boyfriend and a new adventure. The second thing was easier to arrange than the first. She reckons once men found out what she'd done in rowing the Atlantic, they thought she was either out of their league or completely mad.

Her new adventure was to cycle around the United Kingdom's coastline, close to 7000 kilometres, to clean up 78 beaches. At the same time, I was cycling from John o' Groats to Land's End to raise money for Doddie Weir's foundation. Kiko joined the Doddie ride in Newcastle and tagged along for a while.

She was at the back, struggling to get up the hills, so I drifted to the back also and we started chatting. Back at the hotel later that night, there were some WhatsApp messages flying around about the chocolates we had received. Kiko let it be known that she hadn't received any, so the gentlemanly thing was obviously to hand deliver her some.

As she likes to say: 'I shut the door behind him and never let him out. I got the chocolates and a hairy, rugby-playing New Zealander.'

I returned to New Zealand to see my kids, but I kept in touch with Kiko. I was a bit up and down over this period. There was a lot going on in my head due to my separation from Nat. The fact I had to continue in my role as assistant coach meant my ability to be a father to my kids was severely compromised. I could see a scenario where I faded out of their lives and that was devastating to contemplate. It wasn't a particularly happy time, which Kiko picked up on as we continued to talk.

We arranged to meet in Paris when I returned to France. It should have been this fantastic, romantic getaway in one of the world's great cities, but I had something to tell Kiko and I couldn't find the way to do it. This vagueness hung over everything we did, and I don't think she was particularly impressed. Towards the end of the weekend, she finally said something about me not being the same person she'd met. I finally spoke the unspeakable.

'I have to be honest with you. When I leave you here, I'm returning to Pau to go to court where I'm pleading guilty to domestic violence charges. I've spent the weekend dreading having to tell you that.'

Just saying the words out loud was jarring for me. God knows what they sounded like to Kiko. She'd been waiting a long time to meet somebody she liked with similar interests and outlook on life as her — we'd already told each other we thought we were perfect for each other — and here was the same guy telling her he had hit his wife.

To my huge relief, Kiko took it in her stride. Part of it was probably knowing that I hadn't been away with the fairies all weekend for nothing. Part of it, she says, was because she had hit her partner when she was younger, so had some understanding of how arguments could spin out of control. That didn't make me feel any better about what I had done. Obviously there are significant differences, given the power imbalance between a 120-kilogram ex-All Black prop hitting his diminutive wife compared to a girlfriend hitting her boyfriend in a teenage tiff, but her willingness to forgive me and to try to understand did make me love her all the more.

In May 2019, I had my day in court. Agence France-Presse, one of the world's biggest news agencies, covered the court appearance, so it got extensive coverage around the world. It did not make for comfortable reading.

From the *Stuff* website:

Former All Blacks star Carl Hayman admitted to alcohol problems as he was handed a four-month suspended prison sentence for domestic violence in France.

The 39-year-old appeared in a Pau court on Tuesday facing several counts of violence against his wife between 2016 and 2018.

These include 'a powerful slap' necessitating three days off work.

As well as physical violence Hayman was charged with psychological damage, nuisance calls and insults.

'It's inexcusable. I had a problem with alcohol at the end of my professional playing career,' Hayman said.

The 1.94 m, 120 kg Hayman has been playing and coaching in France since shifting there from England where he played on a high salary after the All Blacks 2007 World Cup disaster.

Hayman was Pau forwards coach in the Top 14 championship until he was sacked in January after allegedly fighting with some of his players.

Hayman's lawyer, Christophe Arcaute, told the court: 'He knows that he committed the irreparable.

'To recognise that he's an alcoholic, to admit his weaknesses in this particular environment, that doesn't happen.

'He is aware that the facts are serious. He is teetotal now.'

That last sentence might have been correct at the time, but I read it now and the sentiment is premature, fanciful even. The idea that I could turn the tap off and lose alcohol as my emotional crutch was attractive, but in my case, it would need to be more than an attractive idea.

* * *

Kiko had to put up with a lot in those early days. It was such a fraught time in my life. I was still living in Pau but had lost my job as forwards coach after the New Year's Eve incident with Whopper and Steffon Armitage. I have nothing but gratitude to Simon Mannix, the head coach, and the people at Pau who employed me and stuck with me well beyond my usefulness, but the divorce between me and professional rugby was long overdue. I was never built for coaching, and by that time, my memory was poor and my ability to process new information was terrible. I was a liability, surviving on my name and reputation alone. Once the 'reputation' part of that equation was tarnished, what did I actually have to offer?

I only ever coached out of necessity, never a love for the job. That would have been obvious to anybody working with me.

Nevertheless, my relationship with Kiko was progressing nicely. We went cycling together for a week. It was fine until the end of the week when she reckons she noticed 'unnecessary' or 'emotional' drinking. During the trip itself, we would go to the pub for a meal and a drink at night and it was literally that: a drink or two with dinner. It wasn't like I was going 10 drinks to her one. But at the end of the week, she noticed that when I got on the train to leave, I was having a beer at nine in the morning. That was a strange thing to process for her. There was nothing untoward all week and yet here we were saying goodbye to each other and I'm doing it with a beer in my hand.

The simple truth is that it had become the only way I knew how to deal — or, more accurately, how not to deal — with uncertainty and confusion. Kiko had already become a stabilising influence on me, but left to my own devices and going back to a place where I had no job and no one, I drank to fill the gap. At this point, I couldn't comprehend what that looked like from her perspective: it was just what I did.

On my fortieth birthday, Kiko and I went to clear out the house at Carqueiranne. Among the many items to pack up and store were my wedding photos. That was a strange day. Happy birthday and all that.

In Kiko's words: 'This whole time I could see this incredibly gentle, sensitive, loving giant, but occasionally the demon would come out and he'd revert to complete emotional retardation. I went and saw *A Star is Born*, the film starring Bradley Cooper as a country singer struggling with his internal demons, and it cut really close to the bone. I never felt unsafe around Carl, but I quickly realised his relationship with alcohol was, literally, toxic.'

At the end of 2019, we came out to New Zealand for a couple of months and ended up staying through a COVID-enforced lockdown. I wanted to move back home, to be near the kids if nothing else, but Kiko was unsure. She'd come to the same conclusion as Nat, and that conclusion was that she wasn't going to live on a dairy farm with me. As much as I loved the idea, she was pretty clear that she didn't think a life of isolation was good for me, and she was 100 per cent certain it wasn't good for her. Kiko wasn't certain about New Zealand (or me) at all, but we were enjoying time with the kids, which was cool, and one day she decided to go paddleboarding in New Plymouth, and rocked up to Chaddy's Charters, down near the port.

'Carl,' she said, 'I know this isn't on your radar, but this business is for sale.'

I liked the look of Chaddy's Charters. I knew it was an iconic local business, and gradually came around to the idea. I knew I wanted to make a life with Kiko and loved being out on the water, so what could go wrong?

Plenty, actually, though I can't blame any of it on Kiko, or the business.

I was off the booze and physically fitter than I'd been in a long time due to my amateur career as an Ironman 'athlete', but I noticed a sharp deterioration in my memory. Kiko didn't notice it initially, because she was always blown away by how I remembered all the names of people down the coast, even people I hadn't seen for 30 years. But those weren't the memories I had trouble accessing. I was forgetting what I was doing 10 minutes ago. I was getting scarily confused and having these out-of-body experiences. I'd find myself driving along the road and suddenly realise I had no idea how I'd got in the car, where I was going, or what the purpose of the trip had been in the first place. It was like I had been asleep and woken to find myself driving along the main street of New Plymouth.

Sometimes Kiko, my family or friends would ask me simple questions and I'd find myself tongue-tied. I knew what I wanted to say, but couldn't find or form the words. I'd always held a sneaky pride that I was a bit quicker than I looked, had a dry sense of humour and could respond with a sharp retort when it was called for, but more and more I was living up to the cliché of being a monosyllabic prop.

I was also suffering headaches that were more frequent and intense. Headaches had been a big part of my life since Toulon, but now they were feeling permanent, a locked-in part of my life. They weren't the fleeting kind, nor were they the kind you could chase away with a couple of paracetamol tablets. They were perhaps easier to explain away than the memory loss or the confusion, because I could point to a neck that was buggered from playing more than 400 first-class, professional games of rugby.

While scrums are a lot safer now than in the 1980s, when there was a spate of serious spinal injuries in the front row, particularly among hookers who were the meat in a prop sandwich, there is no getting away from the fact they are a dangerously unnatural phenomenon. The muscles in the human neck, or cervical spine, are designed to carry the weight of your head, nothing more. They, and the seven cervical vertebrae and discs, did not evolve with the idea of cushioning a scrum with close to three tonnes of force going through it. As a tighthead prop, it felt like all that force was being channelled through my neck.

I'd have needles in my neck to calm the inflammation and my ageing discs were a mess, so it was natural to assume my neck was the root cause of my headaches. But these felt different. There were days when they were unmanageable and my sensitivity to light was increasing. I'd have long periods when I just wanted to sit in the dark with my head in my hands and would get irritable and angry if anything or anyone got in the way of me doing just that.

Kiko was getting more and more concerned about the headaches because of what they did for my mental state. I was also having increasing occurrences of night confusions, or terrors, which were frightening for her to deal with. She was getting more and more insistent that I seek specialist help because it didn't matter if the root cause was psychological or physiological, I couldn't continue on this path.

Genevieve Ocean — my fourth child, and Kiko's first — arrived on the scene in February 2021. It was a bloody difficult birth and Osh emerged into this world very white and very floppy. I dealt with this scare in a way that was both predictable and very typical: I went out and got drunk. I had been 15 months free of booze at that point, but what did that matter when there was a crisis in your life you could blot out for a while? Kiko took it about as well as you'd expect somebody who has gone through such an agonising experience to take it. She should have been totally focused on her newborn, but instead she had another childlike person in her life to deal with.

By now Kiko and my frustration at not being able to get tangible assistance here in New Zealand was reaching boiling point. I can't begin to tell you how frustrating it is to be talked to like you're an idiot. I knew something was wrong with me. I knew my brain wasn't working as it should. I didn't know whether that was a psychiatric or a physiological issue, but nobody seemed interested in finding out, either. There was no urgency. No suggestion I get the latest and best brain scans on the market. No acknowledgement that 400-plus games of professional rugby could have negative brain health consequences. Instead, it was: 'Oh, you're just depressed. Here's some antidepressants.'

The links between contact sport and chronic traumatic encephalopathy were well established in literature by now. The sad cases in American football in particular have been highlighted in the media and there was even a big report into the number of ex-Taranaki rugby players who were living and dying with neurodegenerative disease, but nobody I saw was making any connection between the game I had played for most of my life to the symptoms I was exhibiting. I didn't feel just like a number in the system; I felt like I wasn't even part of the system.

When Alix Popham, a Welshman with no medical expertise dealing with his own life-changing diagnosis, came into my life, it felt like the first time anybody from outside my inner circle was taking my problems seriously. Marginalised by the healthcare system that was supposed to have my best interests at heart from cradle to grave, I instead flew to London, and subsequently Mexico, to try to get to the root of my problems and stymie my deterioration.

The testing there was exhaustive and exhausting. They gave me answers, many of which were unpalatable, unthinkable even. They were non-judgemental.

Here in New Zealand, I feel like I'm a hostage to the Accident Compensation Corporation, commonly known as ACC. After a perfunctory consultation with an ACC-chosen neuropsychologist, it was determined that I had depression and that my left-handedness predisposed me towards mental health issues. I know the left-handed thing is rooted in statistical fact, but the whole process seemed designed to belittle and to minimise the idea that my brain had been exposed to significant, repeated, cumulative trauma during the course of a long career, despite a mountain of evidence showing the links between repeated head knocks and neurodegenerative disease, and CTE in particular.

Call me a conspiracy theorist if you like, but I'm not alone in thinking that there's a lot at stake here, and the longer you can claim the scientific link between head injuries and CTE is incomplete, the better it will be for organisations like New Zealand Rugby and ACC.

So that's where I am now: kicking around New Plymouth. As I put the finishing touches on this book, I'm still shuttling between the call of the sea and the farm, and still forgetting shit. I still want to love and be loved, but maybe I've made that too difficult, and I'm still trying and occasionally failing to be the best dad I can to my four children, Sophie, Taylor, Charlie and Genevieve.

I still go to meetings and try to stay on my meds, but sometimes, yes, I still fuck up.

I played close to 450 games of professional rugby, and a bunch more amateur games as well. If I'd lived a life of blameless excellence, perhaps this would have been a classic rugby biography, with whole chapters dedicated to games won and lost.

If I'd done it all properly, had my career moved in lockstep with others of my generation who tasted World Cup glory and left the sport with unblemished reputations, perhaps I would have signed this off with a dedication to all those I had played with and been coached by.

But although rugby is a big part of my story, it's not the whole story.

I loved rugby. At times I couldn't get enough of it. But it damaged me, too. Rugby gave me confidence and it gave me opportunities, but it also provided me with a front for drinking. It played a role in what Kiko calls my 'emotional retardation'.

When my life started spinning out of control, I wasn't conditioned to tell people how scared and confused I was because I had once been the bloody tighthead prop for the All Blacks.

But if you've got this far, you are starting to know who I am.

I used to play rugby and was quite good at it. I'm a man who hit a woman I loved, the mother of three of my children. I'm a father. I'm a hunter and a fisherman. I'm a hard worker. I'm a kid from a farm and still a wannabe farmer. I'm an alcoholic. I'm brain damaged and sometimes scared, sometimes lonely. I'm loving and loyal. I'm a bit of a mess.

Yeah, I'm all that, but there's one other thing I am...

I'm not without hope.

EPILOGUE

RESCUE III, PT II

ONE OF THE MOST famous lines in New Zealand sport was uttered during Team New Zealand's ill-fated defence of the America's Cup in 2003. After a series of breakages, including a broken mast, across five calamitous races, someone on board, probably skipper Dean Barker, was heard on a sound effects mic uttering the immortal line: 'This fucking boat!'

I can empathise.

I want to love *Rescue III*, but some days she makes it so damn hard.

When I started stripping her back, it soon became obvious that the job was bigger than I anticipated. On the surface she looked like she was doing all right for her 70 years, but under the skirts, there was a bit more going on than I ever expected.

It didn't take me long to realise that when I decided to restore her to somewhere near her former glory, I'd really thrown myself in the deep end. I should have asked around before I started, because everyone I know who has embarked on a similar project now tells me the same thing: take a worst-case scenario for the amount of work you think you'll need to do, then multiply that many times over.

Take the deck, for instance. There were a couple of holes that had been patched over with plywood, but when we cut them out, we realised there were other parts of the deck that were also going soft due to rot. We've ended up taking out all the rot and putting a new 17-millimetre deck over the top of the old stuff.

Even that is largely cosmetic. Don't get me started on all the engine parts that have been taken out, cleaned and revived; all the shafts; all the wiring and all the seals that have been replaced.

There's also the inch and a half of grease and oil that had to be cleaned out of the bilge before we could start putting the engine back in. All the old piping has been taken out and disposed of. We've rebuilt that from scratch.

There's also the small matter of 400 silicon-bonded screws to bolster the integrity of the laminates.

Then there's the outer. We've put a fairing compound that sets like concrete on the hull, a coat of fibreglass and another layer of fairing. Finally, she's got a couple of coats of paint.

It's dirty, monotonous work that can see you caked in a layer of dust one day and trying to get resin out of your hair the next. When that epoxy smell gets into your sinuses, you can walk around for days thinking it's following you everywhere.

When I started the project there was a novelty factor to it. I enjoy working with my hands. I enjoy that sense of starting the day at x and having something to show for it when you get to y, but there were days when it felt not just like I was standing still, but actually going backwards.

I wondered if we were ever going to make it.

Rescue III has provided a frighteningly apt metaphor for where I am in my life at the moment.

I might not have her good looks, but I'm dinged up, requiring a bit more work than I can imagine, but I think I'm worth persevering with. I have a bit more to offer this planet yet, even if it's on terms that I find hard to reconcile with my 'former' life. Two steps forward is just as often followed by two and a half steps back. There are days when I have left the boatshed, unable to cope with the setbacks and the lack of progress, but those setbacks are more about me than they are about the boat.

I have endured some moments of personal difficulty and confusion during this process. At times my sense of self-worth has plummeted. I've had to learn to let go and to recalibrate my expectations.

I struggle with the concept of 'the future'. It's been a weight on my mind, and when I think too much about it, I get scared.

Through the course of my long rugby career — a career I can look back on with pride — I was living life with the accelerator pressed down hard. I played hard, I trained hard, I partied hard. To some extent, that continued post-career. I was always conscious of the next goal, whether it was completing an Ironman, or climbing mountains.

My life was a series of external motivations. I was a doer. I couldn't understand people who let life come to them. I always needed to be chasing something: a trophy of one type or another to put on the mantelpiece.

I can't keep chasing goals now. My body won't let me. Over the past two years, I've noticed a considerable decline, not just in my cognition, but also in my energy levels. Like an iPhone, my battery drains quickly and needs constant recharging. That's when I get angry with *Rescue III*, when I feel I should be doing more, when I know that not long ago, I would have done plenty more, but after a couple of hours, my focus goes and I shut down. That can make me irrationally angry with myself.

I need to learn to be happy being, not doing. I have to be more present in the moment, not looking for the next external goal.

Kiko has a great outlook on it. She says the future is about trying to find the beauty in every day. That there's no point worrying about what I might be like tomorrow, because that will only end up ruining today. She's right, of course. With every fibre of my being, I know she's right, but the mind can be a dangerous tool when it's got time on its hands and it starts to wander.

Some days, those simple ideas get away from me and I start to despair. I want to be in the present. I want to be a great father to my four kids, whom I love more than I can explain, but the thought that I might end up being a burden to them scares the hell out of me.

I spent the bulk of my career with the idea of providing for my family, for securing our future. That's why I found it easier than most to give up on the black jersey and take a different path. Now I know it's not about what I can provide, but just about being present. I don't have to smash myself to bits for anybody now.

If you read this book with a certain mindset, you could be left with the impression that my life, particularly my post-playing life, has been a journey linking one set of unfortunate events to another.

I try to look at it another way. Remember right back to the start, living and working in Pau. Those were my darkest days, right?

I committed a dreadful act of violence on my wife, an act that was the precursor to separation and divorce. I had fallen out of love with professional rugby and knew I didn't want to be part of the machinery any longer. My drinking went from unhealthy to dangerous. I was struggling emotionally and cognitively and fighting back suicidal ideation on a daily basis. I had a fight with two of my friends that precipitated me being sacked from my job.

It was a dire time in my life and yet I can look at the green shoots that emerged out of the deepening cracks in my life.

For a start, I sought help for my alcohol dependency. My road to sobriety has been potholed and imperfect, but admitting a problem to my family and friends broke down the bullshit macho image that had constrained me. Once you stop having to be the hard man, you can admit to how fragile you really are. I can talk about problems that I once would have been ashamed of and I'm getting better at asking for help.

My life is not without sunshine, nor is it without hope. I've been lucky to have been able to get specialist treatment in Mexico, and to be part of a drug trial that I hope will lead to big breakthroughs in the ability to fight back the march of dementia. Every month, there seems to be positive news from the medical science community about the progress fighting insidious neurodegenerative diseases.

I'm glad I'm out of rugby, now, but I don't hate the sport. I'd be quite happy if any of my kids wanted to play the game, although the sport's leaders still need to have urgent conversations about the volume of rugby and the way it is played now, with the men's game in particular moving from collision to collision between fitter, bigger and stronger athletes. Rugby gave me so much, not just materially, but in terms of understanding concepts like camaraderie and teamwork.

It's been teamwork that has got *Rescue III* over the line and that has enabled us to relaunch a vessel that should serve the New Plymouth and Taranaki tourism community for another 70 years. It has taken a small village to re-raise a boat.

There's Brian 'Chook' Fowler, an 85-year-old former dairy farmer who comes in most days to help out. He's a wonderful guy who was happy if I brought him a bit of beef from the farm from time to time, or let him come out with me to check my crayfish pots.

Chris Powell is a former commercial fisherman and builder. He claims he's never been a boatbuilder, but he knows his way around *Rescue III* better than me. He came in expecting a quick two- or three-day project and was still coming in five months later.

There's the kid, Roger, a 16-year-old who loves working on engines. My uncle, Lee Drummond, who owns a marine services company, was a huge help, as were other local fibreglass and paint businesses.

That old boat, beaten up and in need of an overhaul, is a good example of what can happen if you surround yourself with good people.

There's a lesson in that.

I'm not the same person I was as a carefree kid, whose idea of heaven was camping down the back of the farm by the creek with an iron plate, a box of matches and a packet of sausages. I'm not the same person I was when I was a young, impressionable footy player trying to master the arcane arts of tighthead prop. I'm certainly not the same person I was when I was an All Black, or when I was propping up clubs in the two richest domestic leagues in the world.

Shit, I'm not the same person I was two years ago, before my diagnosis.

But I'm still Carl Hayman, and that was my story.

AFTERWORD

THE HAPPIEST I'VE SEEN Carl Hayman is in the shed at the old family farm in Oaonui, a windswept patch of soil, sand and green, green grass just out of Ōpunake on State Highway 45, or the Surf Highway, as it has been remarketed to attract those in search of the perfect break.

From the rear of the property, you look out to the Tasman Sea and the Maui gas fields. From the front, your eyes skip the rich pastures and are drawn to the maunga, Mount Taranaki, its conical shape interrupted only by the proud protrusion that is Fanthams Peak. There, in one 360-degree sweep, is Taranaki at its most elemental: the oil and gas industry, the iron-sand coastline, dairy farms, the mountain and the surrounding national park.

If there's one other thing that Taranaki locals like to be known for, it's producing tough rugby players.

In this shed, among the usual detritus you might find on a farm, including ride-on mowers, a welding machine, fencing wire and every other tool you might conceivably need, there are a bunch of nondescript boxes that constitute the career of, by general consensus, one of the finest tighthead props ever to grace a rugby field.

Not that Carl would describe himself this way. At his most ebullient, his cockiest, perhaps, you might get a wry smile and a concession that: 'I went okay, yeah.' But the praise would soon be shifted to others — coaches, teammates, even opposition players that taught him the ropes.

It's a modesty we associate not just with prop forwards, but also those brought up on the land. Farmers don't like to get ahead of themselves. They know how quickly a good year can be followed by a bad one. They're reluctant spenders. Taranaki is home to some of the most productive dairy land in the country and some of the most modest farmhouses.

'Do you know what I like about being down here?' Carl says at one point. 'Things don't really change.'

Stability is going to be increasingly important for Carl as he gets older. So are memories. Here in this shed — and a good shed is prized more highly than an ensuite and walk-in wardrobe around these parts — the boxes contain jerseys, rugby balls from big games and, most remarkably, a video of every televised game he played in New Zealand. The containers also contain folders full of clippings and relevant sports collections. One immediately catches my eye. It was a special lift-out insert previewing the Lions tour in 2005, which was folded into the *Herald on Sunday*.

The weatherproofing and temperature inside that shed must have been similar to the Smithsonian, because the magazine, despite being produced on newsprint stock, was crisp, dry and beautifully preserved. I started riffling through the pages, jogging my memory, until I stopped on page 15.

On the left-hand side of the page was half of Shane Williams' face, with a 300-word column from sports funny man James McOnie telling us why we should love the diminutive Welsh wing. On the right-hand side was a column by this writer, telling Lions supporters why they should love an unbearded and reasonably fresh-faced young Highlanders prop called Carl Hayman.

'Because he's what New Zealanders used to be like before pubs started calling themselves bars and farmers swapped Land Rovers for 4x4s with coffee-cup holders,' I wrote. 'Because by the time he was 23, he looked 36. Because when people talk about heartland (he was born in Ōpunake and raised in Taranaki and Otago) they are referring to people like him...

'Hayman is an unreconstructed outdoors man — shooting, fishing and rugby will always take precedence over a couscous salad and a latte with new friends at a trendy cafe. It's nice to know there are a few of them still around.

'Hayman, the 1000th All Black and one you've got to love.'

All fairly glib, page-filling stuff, and the truth was that I didn't know Carl from a bar of industrial-strength soap back then. While I covered the All Blacks regularly and had a couple of overseas World Cup campaigns (2003 and 2007) on my resumé, I was never lead rugby writer for the papers I worked on. Hand on heart, I can say I preferred it that way. Cricket was my first and strongest sporting love, and while for a time the Black Caps' environment was a hive of backbiting, suspicion and underperformance, I found the characters who played cricket more interesting and three-dimensional.

To me, Carl was just another unknowable All Black to be written about more as myth than man. It would be fair to say he preferred it that way as well. While the consensus was that he was a 'good bugger', he wasn't a noted raconteur in front of the cameras or a line of dictaphones (which was a shame, really, because when you talked to his teammates, they made a point of saying what a quick and dry sense of humour he possessed). It was a source of some amusement when news of Carl's burgeoning relationship with TVNZ reporter Natalie Crook started to emerge — Carl had seemingly gone from zero to 100 pretty quickly when it came to media relations.

The sense of mystery was only amplified when the prop packed his bags and left New Zealand following the disastrous 2007 World Cup campaign, despite having been one of the few to enhance his reputation. He did so in part to escape the claustrophobia of being an All Black, but mostly he did so to secure his and his family's future. He'd watched his mum and dad try and fail — through no fault of their own — to become farm owners, and he'd watched them grow apart as a result. He became, probably, the highest-paid player in the world when he signed for Newcastle, but not everything was as it seems, as you'll have learned in these pages.

Like most rugby fans, I expected we would see the name 'Hayman' return to the black jersey once he'd made a bit of cash, in time for the 2011 World Cup on home soil. It nearly happened, but as the negotiations got to the sharp end, a piece of widely disseminated misinformation was enough for Carl to decide he was better off overseas.

When Carl's and my professional life collided in 2021, one of the first things he said to me was that if he had his time again, he would have retired after the '07 World Cup. He said it with such conviction that I believed him, but the warmth with which he talked about his time in Toulon, in particular, means I'm no longer so sure.

We connected through a sad story. His story. For some years now, I have been reporting on neurodegenerative diseases in retired rugby players and the links with the repetitive head injuries they suffered while playing. I had heard from multiple sources that Carl was struggling with certain aspects of his life and had read the reports of his domestic assault conviction in France. Initially, he expressed little interest in joining a lawsuit being filed against World Rugby and some of its constituent boards, or even in undergoing clinical testing that could determine why his life had started to spiral.

With encouragement and support from former counterparts who were going through similar challenges, Carl not only received the diagnosis that will, in part, dictate his remaining years, but also agreed to sit down with me and tell his story. The story appeared on my Substack, *The Bounce*, and *The Spinoff* website simultaneously. The impact was immediate and at a speed neither of us had anticipated. It started to reverberate around the world, being picked up everywhere, from giant UK publications *The Guardian* and *Daily Mail* and global news agency Reuters to all the major Australian news outlets, and even places like CNN, for which rugby has never been a major feature.

Carl's disarming honesty was a pleasant surprise. Although he had to be a little careful about what he said due to being party to an impending lawsuit, nothing was out of bounds.

'In hindsight, as much as I enjoyed it at the time, I don't think [playing rugby] week after week for 10 months of the year did much good for me. At the time I felt indestructible,' he told me. 'I never got injured, I trained bloody hard. I literally felt that I was indestructible, but if I knew then what I know

now, I don't think I would have played post the 2007 World Cup. I think I would have stopped playing.'

This was remarkable to me. Of all the men — and they are all men — who I have talked to who have been afflicted by this disease and who trace it back to their playing careers, virtually all of them felt the need to point out they wouldn't have traded rugby for a better later life. Carl was the first dissenter.

'I'm 41. I've still got a massive part of my life ahead of me, and when you live with something like this, it certainly makes every day a challenge.'

Every day has been a challenge. Sometimes he wins, sometimes, as you've read, the days get the better of him. There is a searing honesty to Carl that can make for uncomfortable listening and, I hope, has made for uncomfortable reading. There was nothing inauthentic about him, as he recounted his life, from an idyllic upbringing on a farm in his beloved coastal Taranaki, to his conversion from an average lock to a preternaturally talented tighthead prop, to his relatively short and star-crossed All Blacks career, a life as a well-paid professional pioneer, his battles with alcohol, a failed marriage, new love, diagnosis and a future that is full of uncertainty and yet not without optimism.

I started this winding road as the journalist with Carl as the subject, but like most people who get sucked into Carl's orbit, I now consider him a friend.

Some days I worry about my new mate. Some days he worries about himself too. But I've yet to catch up with him without him greeting me with a big smile on his face, a firm handshake and a cheerful: 'Shit, we've got a bit to talk about today.'

Long after this book sits forgotten on the shelves, I hope that will continue.

– Dylan Cleaver, November 2022

ACKNOWLEDGEMENTS

I would like to thank the publishers and in particular Alex Hedley for the opportunity to write this book. It's an honest representation of my life and career I will always be grateful for.

In Dylan Cleaver I found someone I could be open with and talk about my thoughts in a reflective way. That was special and I thank him for his honesty and dedication to the book.

I was concerned about how this book might impact my kids, but I hope that it gives them inspiration and resilience for their lives ahead. Life is not always easy. Sometimes we need to ask for help.